YOUR HEART
YOUR PLANET

Thank you for caring.

Harry Diamond

YOUR HEART
YOUR PLANET

by

Harvey Diamond

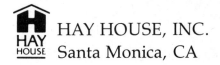
HAY HOUSE, INC.
Santa Monica, CA

YOUR HEART YOUR PLANET
by Harvey Diamond

Library of Congress Catalog Card No. 90-80650

Library of Congress Cataloging-in-Publication Data

Diamond, Harvey, 1945–
    Your heart, your planet by Harvey Diamond.
        p.   cm.
    Includes bibliographical references.
        ISBN 0-937611-95-6 : $16.95.—ISBN 0-937611-96-4 (pbk.) : $10.00
        1. Nutrition.   2. Coronary heart disease—Prevention.   3. Man—
    Influence on environment.   4. Food habits.   I. Title.
    RA784.D52   1990
    304.2—dc20   90-80650
                                                                            CIP

90 91 92 93 94 95   10 9 8 7 6 5 4 3 2 1
First Printing, May 1990

Published and Distributed in the United States by
Hay House, Inc.
501 Santa Monica Boulevard
Post Office Box 2212
Santa Monica, California 90406 USA

Printed in the United States of America

DEDICATION

This book is dedicated to

FRANCISCO "CHICO" MENDES,

who was born and raised in the Amazon rain forests of Brazil. He struggled to preserve his beloved forests from decimation by cattle ranchers. He was murdered for his efforts on December 22, 1988. He was 44 years old.

A SPECIAL NOTE

Thank you for purchasing this book. In so doing, you have made a contribution to the healing of our environment. Your purchase will enable the FIT FOR LIFE Foundation to fund projects such as tree planting, land reclamation, education, and other efforts essential to the future of our planet.

TABLE OF CONTENTS

ACKNOWLEDGEMENTS

I wish to thank the most loving and caring person I have ever known—my wife, Marilyn—whose dedication and commitment to healing is an inspiration to anyone who has ever met her.

Special thanks also to Chuck Ashman, not only an advisor and manager of unparalleled excellence, but also a true and dear friend who is always there.

Thank you, John Robbins, for being the caring person that you are; for putting your concern for our planet and our children before your own personal needs; for opening my understanding to the seriousness of this subject.

Thank you, Robin Hur—a person entirely committed to the healing of our planet. Your tireless efforts in researching and chronicling the forces that impact the environment of our Earth have made you one of the most knowledgeable people on this subject in the world.

Thank you, Beau, Lisa, and Greg, my children, for whom this work is given meaning.

And thank you everyone at Hay House, especially Andrew Ettinger, Linda Tomchin, and Louise Hay, for having the concern, passion, and dedication necessary to bring this book to the public's attention.

INTRODUCTION

It can be said with a fair degree of certainty that, given the opportunity to have any three wishes granted, most of us, along with vast wealth and un-limited power, would request vibrant, glorious health. In fact, of what value would the first two gifts be, if the lucky recipient were too unhealthy to enjoy them?

Who among us is **not** interested in his or her health? No one wishes to be sick or to become a medical statistic. For ourselves and for our loved ones, we all feel a deep-seated desire to experience boundless, energetic health.

In assessing your health, there are two factors that are so closely interconnected and inseparable that they both must be taken into consideration: your own personal level of well-being, and the well-being of planet Earth—which is, in reality, your life-support system. There is no difference whatsoever between being kept alive in a hospital, hooked up to the most technologically advanced life-support equipment available, and the life you presently en-joy, provided to you by our planet.

The three most urgent and necessary prerequisites of life are air, water, and food. They are all gifts to us from our planet, so in no way am I speaking figuratively when I say that planet Earth is your—**our**—life-support system. At a conference on healing the planet organized by the UCLA School of Medicine, it was noted that "taking responsibility for your personal health must now include understanding the environmental forces that adversely affect your well-being."*

Imagine this unfortunate scenario, if you will. Someone very dear to you is hospitalized and totally dependent on life-support equipment for survival. When you go to visit this person who means so much to you, you are astonished to see that the equipment that stands between the life and death of your loved one is an absurdly inefficient hodgepodge of used washing machine parts, old levers and pulleys, and bits and pieces of broken-down machinery, choking and chugging along like a discordant four-piece band falling down a flight of stairs. Just when this jumble of patchwork machine

---

*"Our Common Future: Healing the Planet," symposium organized by the UCLA School of Medicine in cooperation with Physicians for Social Responsibility and the Beyond War Foundation, May 13, 1989.

parts seems to be coughing its way to its last gasp, a big, slovenly, cigarette-smoking attendant invades the room, and with one thunderous blow, kicks the faltering equipment into further activity. He then disappears from the room as abruptly as he entered, leaving behind a cloud of body odor and deadly tobacco smoke. Are there even words to describe the outrage you would feel at that moment?

The fact is, if a dear one, or you yourself, had to rely on a life-support system, you would want to be totally confident that it was working meticulously well and that whoever was in charge of overseeing its activities was the most highly qualified and dedicated person available. Does the life-support system that we are all inextricably connected to deserve any less concern and attention? Hardly. Yet, as you are reading this, the stewardship of our great and glorious planet Earth is on a collision course. As we increasingly use and abuse our planet, deplete and poison the soil, cut down trees, pollute the air and water, and plunder other resources, we have begun to bear the repercussions of these activities. Aren't we all aware of the greenhouse effect? Of global warming? Of the hole in the ozone layer that protects us from harmful ultraviolet rays? What about the billions of pounds of toxins that are being dumped into the land and water and pumped into the air? We know that carbon dioxide levels from the burning of fossil fuels are increasing at an alarming rate, while trees that eliminate carbon dioxide are being cut down at a record pace.

The environment of Earth, which is virtually our life-support system, is gasping and pleading for help, crying out to us the only way it can. To ignore that fact or to busy ourselves exclusively with other matters, hoping that more concerned and committed citizens will deal with the crisis before it's too late would be like seeing a loved one in the predicament described above and not registering a complaint or taking any action. To do nothing is to commit a slow suicide, condemning our children to an uncertain future that they would have to deal with, even though they had no hand in its creation.

Before this starts to sound like a morose, doomsday depiction of what life has in store for us if changes are not made, let me assure you that **that** is not what this little book is about. Quite the opposite is true. We **are** at a crossroad, most assuredly, but the situation is such that we are **not** beyond the point of no return. Far from it. Not that we can afford to ignore our situation and hope that it will correct itself. We can't and it won't. However, the remedy is surprisingly attainable. The dimensions of the problem might make it appear insurmountable to some, but there are measures that are remarkably easy to employ and just as effective. It's simply a matter of having the information and then acting on it. There is something that **you** personally can do. In fact, without you, there's little hope of success.

Let me ask you a hypothetical question. Suppose you were driving near the outskirts of town on your way to an important meeting, and you saw a brushfire in the hills moving rapidly towards the city. Also suppose you were absolutely the only person on this stretch of highway. Would you continue on your present course and hope that the fire department would be called in time to avert a real tragedy, or would you leave the highway, find a phone, and **make sure** that the proper authorities were advised of the situation?

When you look at how little effort would have to be expended to avoid what could escalate into a real catastrophe, it hardly seems possible that you would not opt to make that call to the fire department. This scenario can be likened to what we are facing in terms of rescuing our planet from further distress so that we and our children can enjoy a more promising future. A very slight effort on your part can make a significant contribution to the healing of our life-support system, **and** it will also improve your own personal health.

If it is true that a minor, almost inconsequential effort on your part will indeed bring about noticeable and meaningful results, is there anything that could possibly **prevent** you from playing a role in such a worthy and lofty endeavor?

When we look at the vast, multifaceted subject of health and all of its many levels of relevance that have a bearing on our well-being, and add to that the voluminous body of information pertaining to the effect of human life on the environment, we are dealing with a mass of data so immense and far-reaching that it stuns the intellect. So we might expect that a book discussing these subjects **and** the partial resolution of the predicament would be too heavy to lift! Yet you are holding in your hand a book that tackles the problem, promises so much, and is of such modest dimensions. How can that be?

When I began to address the mammoth amount of data on our environmental crisis, I realized that it would simply be an exercise in futility to attempt to cover all of it in this book. Such extensive coverage would be too laborious and discouraging for the average individual, who, for the most part, is looking for **simple** answers to complicated issues.

Presently, there is no shortage of doom-and-gloom predictions about what is in store for us. Some are indeed frightening, but I don't want you to think that this book falls into that category. It does not. Yes, it gives a description of the status of our planet and points out some possible consequences of continued neglect and abuse. But more importantly, it is a message full of promise, encouragement, and optimism. I could not disagree more with those who say it's too late, that there is no hope. It is **never** too late. There is **always** hope. Healing is every bit as much a part of life on Earth as is any other phenomenon. And **healing will proceed as required**. We—you and I—are in the grand position of assisting in that healing process.

With this knowledge in mind, my task was clear. I **knew** that people were concerned, of that there was no doubt. Most people I know who were shown how they could help, jumped for the opportunity to do so, given the magnitude of the consequences of doing nothing. It became my goal to set forth a formula, easily understood and easily put into practice, that would produce the greatest results, with the least amount of effort, in the shortest period of time.

Thus, what I offer you is a two-fold opportunity:

1. To quickly obtain an awareness of the need to heal our Earth—an issue that is of such critical significance to all of us.

2. To take a course of action which, although requiring only a minimal amount of your energy, will bring about increased health and vitality for you and your loved ones, and effect positive results on a global level.

We all have a grand opportunity to participate in a truly restorative effort on behalf of Mother Nature. It will take a concerted effort from **everyone** concerned. Because of the tremendous need for corrective measures **now**, it is essential that we don't lose sight of the goal by pointing fingers of blame at yesterday's shortsightedness or by creating factions that are at odds with one another. Doing so could lead to useless accusations and fruitless violence, two indulgences that are totally counterproductive and that only serve to undermine the objective.

If someone throws a rock at you, what do you do? Don't you move farther away from that person so as not to be hit? In this undertaking, we cannot afford to move farther away from each other. We all need to work together—which precludes divisive activities that focus attention on individual differences rather than on solutions. This is not a time for conflict. It is a time for compromise and cooperation. It is not a time for hostility. It is a time for healing and harmony.

Thank you for taking the time.

Thank you for caring.

Harvey Diamond

PART I

The Dilemma

DEAR HEART

What is that special, endearing term we use with those we cherish?

"Sweetheart."

How do we express ourselves when we want to go directly to an important point without wasting time?

"Let's get to the heart of the matter."

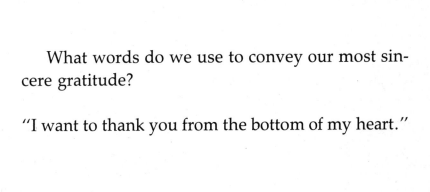

What words do we use to convey our most sincere gratitude?

"I want to thank you from the bottom of my heart."

"I love you with all my heart" is one way to describe how much we love someone.

Every year on one of our favorite national holidays, people all over the country send endearing messages to those they love—to their sweethearts. It's called Valentine's Day and its symbol is the heart. A fitting symbol it is! When you look at the human heart and its pumping and circulatory system of arteries and vessels, you see an instrument of inexplicable **precision**, **complexity**, and **perfection**. The heart is a fist-sized marvel of construction that performs continuously, **nonstop**, 24 hours a day for decades on end—for a century or more, if need be.

Viewed with awe by those who study it, the heart is a masterpiece of strength and endurance. It must be to beat approximately 100,000 times a day, every day.

Beating steadily two-and-a-half billion times in a lifetime . . . pumping an average of six quarts of blood through 96,000 miles of blood vessels every minute!

That is the equivalent of more than 25,000 quarts pumped every day or more than half a billion quarts in a lifetime.

Life itself depends on the constant flow of that river of life, the blood.

Every organ, every **cell** of your body, is bathed, cleansed, and nourished by the bloodstream that is pumped by the heart.

If any part of your body were not provided with oxygen by the blood, it would quickly wither and die.

So magnificent is the heart and its pumping system that scientists with the most sophisticated technology available to them have been totally unsuccessful in their attempts to duplicate it. The heart has valves thinner than tissue paper, which are sturdier than steel.

When surgeons replace heart valves with silicone parts, the hard, man-made materials become battered and lose their shape after only a few years.

But the delicate, durable tissues of a healthy heart exert their force and withstand the beating for a lifetime.

And we all have one of these miracle machines beating away in our chests, giving us life.

Any effort you make to protect and strengthen your heart is time well spent. But, alas, our hearts—yours, your parents', your children's, **all** of our hearts—are under siege.

A battle is being waged against our hearts, and the enemy is gaining an upper hand.

This will continue only if **we** allow it to.

We can stop it and we can stop it **right now!**

What is this dreadful enemy and how do we prevail over it?

ATHER-O...WHAT?

First, the villain, bent on destroying our hearts: **atherosclerosis.**

That's the big, unwieldy word you have undoubtedly heard but may not understand completely. Remember, our bodies have 96,000 miles of arteries and veins supplying oxygenated blood to every cell.

In its most simple definition, atherosclerosis is the clogging, narrowing, and closing of these arteries. When the arteries providing blood to the heart muscles are closed, the result is a heart attack and the likelihood of death due to what is called coronary heart disease.

When the arteries to the brain are blocked, the result is a stroke. When we add up all the deaths in the United States that can be attributed to the effects of all cardiovascular diseases, we find that nearly one million people die every year because of it.[1]

About every 35 seconds, day and night, **24 hours a day, someone dies due to this condition.**[2] This statistic says that cardiovascular disease is much more than just the number-one cause of death in our country. If you add up **all** other causes of death by disease—cancer, lung disease, diabetes—**all diseases combined**—they would not come close to equaling the deaths from atherosclerosis/cardiovascular disease alone.[3]

In fact, so prevalent is this problem in our country that one shocking study tells us that a deplorable **98 percent of our children already have at least one symptom of heart disease.**[4]

So, how do we deal with atherosclerosis? What actually causes it, and how do we protect ourselves from it? Perhaps you will be surprised to learn that **atherosclerosis is almost always completely and totally within our control.**

IT'S NO MYSTERY

Atherosclerosis is not "caught" or "accidental," nor is it in any way a mystery. All of the latest, most comprehensive medical research of the most rigorous nature—the most advanced medical knowledge in history—has made it absolutely clear that diets high in saturated fat and cholesterol produce atherosclerosis, which results in heart disease and strokes.

This information bears even more impact when we learn that of the 2.1 million deaths from the 10 leading causes in the United States, diet plays a role in a full 65 percent. If you discount deaths from suicide and unintentional injuries such as auto accidents, the percentage of deaths that feature diet as a contributing factor is closer to 75 percent!

What foods will help lower this awesome percentage?

Fruits, vegetables, and whole grains.

What foods are primarily responsible for this saturated fat and cholesterol that is clogging our arteries and killing us? The research again tells us: animal products (meat, chicken, fish, dairy products, and eggs).

The evidence is in. It is overwhelming. It is undeniable. It is absolute and it is impressive.

The more fruits, vegetables, and whole grains you eat, the lower will be your risk of clogged arteries.

The more animal products you eat, the more likely you are to die of the effects of atherosclerosis. Period. No doubt about it!

HELP FROM THE GOOD GUYS

So obvious is the link between animal products and atherosclerosis that on October 7th, 1988, we received the most timely and convincing verification of the need to reduce our intake of animal products when the nation's top medical doctor, the United States Surgeon General, Dr. C. Everett Koop, released the "Report on Nutrition and Health."

This highly comprehensive report, based on over 2,000 scientific research studies, left no doubt that our standard meat-based, fat-laden American diet is, in Dr. Koop's words, "killing millions prematurely and ruining the lives of tens of millions."

The report established as **national policy** a reduction in the consumption of animal products, with a simultaneous increase in fruits, vegetables, and grains.

And then, in what would seem to underscore most emphatically the Surgeon General's landmark report, the National Research Council, the working arm of the National Academy of Sciences, released its own dietary guidelines in March of 1989. It marked the first time ever that the Council made such definitive dietary recommendations. Their committee of experts took three years to examine nearly **6,000** studies and to compile a 1,400-page report. Not surprisingly, the report echoes the recommendations of the Surgeon General.

AND THE VERDICT IS . . .

The same conclusion has been reached by the National Cancer Institute.

The American Heart Association.

The World Health Organization.

And virtually every other health-related institution in the United States.

Even the government's National Institute of Health, recognizing that the debate over whether diet actually has an effect on blood cholesterol levels and life expectancy, has released its recommendations. The Institute states that "the relationship between high blood cholesterol and heart disease was undisputed and that there were unequivocal benefits to reducing blood cholesterol levels."[4A]

Even a slight increase in your consumption of fruit, vegetables, and whole grains, and a slight reduction in your consumption of animal products, gives you a significant measure of protection against atherosclerosis.

EDUCATION OR INDOCTRINATION?

What a revelation this must be for so many people! Especially since we have collectively been bombarded by propaganda imploring us to consume increasing quantities of animal products—**for health**, of all things.

I remember, as a child in grade school, those impressive, full-color charts heralding the importance of the four food groups—two of which were saturated fat- and cholesterol-laden meat and dairy products. Now I discover that those charts were supplied by the National Dairy Council! What better place to indoctrinate an impressionable child than in the classroom where reading and writing are being taught!

Today, as an adult, I see television picking up where the classroom leaves off. Slick, expensively produced commercials try to sell us on ideas like "beef is real food for real people."

What does that make people who don't eat meat? Androids? There are ads for the "incredible edible egg," and commercials telling us that "milk is good for every body." And, unfortunately, in the past, we have succumbed all too easily to this advertising propaganda, obediently gobbling up our "protein" and milk every day.

Now, in the aftermath of all the scientific campaigns to convince us to reduce our intake of animal products in order to lower our incidence of heart disease, we see the commercials for what they really are: obvious attempts to raise industry profits, at the expense of our health **and** the health of our children. Every day more and more of us are waking up to this exploitation.

In this society, where eating animal products has become a **way of life**, we now know from our scientific and medical researchers that our love affair with animal products is actually a **way of death**.

PASS (ON) THE CHOLESTEROL, PLEASE

Over the last few years, an awareness of cholesterol and its harm to our diets has certainly come to light in a big way. Books abound on the subject, and shopping malls and airports even have stands set up where you can get your cholesterol level tested. People are concerned about its role in heart disease, so they are making every effort to reduce their cholesterol levels.

CHOLESTEROL DOESN'T GROW ON TREES

There is still some confusion, however, about where cholesterol is actually found.

Allow me to put this confusion to rest for you once and forever. Cholesterol is produced in the liver and cells of animals and **nowhere else in the Universe**.

That's not opinion or speculation, either. That's fact. Whatever you're eating—if it didn't have a liver, it cannot contain cholesterol! In other words, it is impossible to ingest cholesterol when you are eating foods that come from the plant kingdom.

Surprisingly, I am frequently asked, "What about avocados?" I always answer by posing the question, "Do avocados have livers?" There is simply **no** cholesterol to be found in anything that grows from the ground.

You can eat fruits, vegetables, and grains to your heart's content and be safe in the knowledge that you are not taking in even **one** milligram of cholesterol.

The one and only source of cholesterol is, of course, animal products.

And the reason that cholesterol has become such a hot item of discussion is because of our overconsumption of **all** animal products. The formula for reducing the level of cholesterol in your blood is a simple one:

Reduce your animal products consumption!

This knowledge will help you prevent the number-one cause of death—heart disease.

It will also help you lower your risk of the number-two cause of death—cancer.

In mid-1989, the American Cancer Society announced plans to undertake the most extensive and expensive research study in history to provide the link between diet and cancer. Including 50 million people in its survey, at a cost of $126 million, it is seeking to firmly substantiate that the incidence of cancer can be cut in half in the next 15 to 20 years if, in addition to reducing smoking and alcohol consumption, people will also "drastically cut down on intake of fat and drastically increase intake of vegetables."[5]

YOU HAVE A CHOICE

When you consider that we are being universally encouraged to **increase** our intake of foods high in fiber and complex carbohydrates, and to **decrease** our intake of foods high in saturated fat and cholesterol, it is an absurdity that we still eat more animal products than any other food. Animal products are not only extremely high in saturated fat and cholesterol, but they are also virtually **devoid** of fiber and complex carbohydrates. In other words, they could not be in more direct opposition to what is being recommended.

Taking drugs and eating oat bran every day without other dietary changes is merely masking the problem. To continue eating large quantities of animal products while trying to reduce the resulting cholesterol level with drugs and oats is like locking your garage door **after** your car has been stolen.

The way to lower the level of cholesterol in your blood, or to prevent it from ever becoming a problem, is to eat fewer animal products. Just check the 1988 Surgeon General's Report on Health and Nutrition.

In all likelihood, this information will be quite surprising to many. What will come as an even greater surprise is that the reduction of animal products in your diet will not only benefit you personally, but will also bring about some profound changes in areas where you just might not have expected them.

THE BIG PICTURE

As is true in the universe, the microcosm imitates the macrocosm. What is happening to us as individuals is also happening to our planet in its entirety. Our obsessive appetite for animal products is not only wreaking havoc with our personal health, but it is taking its toll on our planet's health as well.

IS IT GETTING HOT IN HERE?

You are probably aware of the growing concern over the global warming caused by the "greenhouse effect."

That concern is most assuredly justified. Never before in the history of the world have people actually had to be anxious or fearful about the state of the atmosphere of Earth.

There is a delicate balance that must constantly be maintained. Earth's atmosphere has just the right amount of carbon dioxide for life to flourish. Carbon, which is stored in the Earth, is continuously recycled through the land, the oceans, and the atmosphere. Changes in carbon dioxide levels bring about changes in the climate.

Earth's climate is maintained **only** when the amount of energy from the sun absorbed by the planet **equals** the amount returned to space. This is determined by the amount of carbon dioxide in the atmosphere. If it were not for carbon dioxide trapping enough warmth, the heat from the sun would merely reflect off the Earth, leaving the planet too cold to be inhabited.

For hundreds of millions of years, the proper balance of carbon dioxide has been maintained by nature to provide Earth with just the right temperature to allow life to be lived in comfort. However, technological advances have now provided the means for upsetting nature's fragile equilibrium. So much, in fact, that it is affecting that delicate balance.

Since the advent of the Industrial Revolution, unprecedented amounts of carbon dioxide have been released into the atmosphere through the burning of fossil fuels, oil, gas, and coal.

The build-up of carbon dioxide has reached such a staggering level that it is actually retarding the escape of solar energy into space. It can be likened to a blanket over the Earth. The heat comes in and can't get out. So, precisely like a greenhouse, Earth's lower atmosphere is heating up. This build-up of carbon dioxide can be compared to the closed windows of a car left out in the sun. They let the heat of the sun in, but not out.

Unfortunately, this warming of the planet doesn't just allow for more days at the beach. Rather, it carries with it some potentially catastrophic repercussions. Droughts could not only become more frequent, but also more lengthy and severe. Ask anyone living in the American grain belt, which was scorched by a record drought in 1988, if things don't seem to be heating up. The 1980s saw five of the hottest years in recorded history.[6]

ICE IS NICE

Most of the Antarctic continent is covered by ice nearly two miles thick. These truly massive ice sheets help to cool the Earth by reflecting sunlight back into space like a mirror. If the glaciers shrink, more sunlight will hit the Earth, further heating the planet.

The Arctic icecap in an area north of Greenland that plays the crucial role of reflecting 80 percent of incoming solar radiation back into space, shrank by 30 percent from 1976 to 1987.[7]

The Ross Ice Shelf is a floating slab of ice the size of France that acts as a barrier to hold back the huge mass of ice that covers West Antarctica. Warming could cause the shelf's leading edge to disintegrate and destroy the barrier that contains the unstable West Antarctic ice sheet behind it. If West Antarctica's ice sheet collapses and melts, it could cause the sea level to rise some 20 feet. Flooding would become commonplace. Even a small increase in the sea level could wreak havoc. Storm surges would threaten coastlines more and more frequently.

IS IT TOO LATE TO ACT?

Coastal commissions in Maine, Massachusetts, Maryland, Florida, North and South Carolina, Louisiana, Oregon, Washington, and California have already begun to incorporate sea-level rise measures into coastal planning.[8]

London has already installed a barrier across the Thames River to protect itself from tidal surges that threaten that city even now.

In 1989, the National Oceanographic and Atmospheric Administration, as well as two University of Toronto scientists, announced, **independently**, that the world's oceans have been warming and rising twice as fast as previously observed.[9] Like any other material, oceans expand; water rises as it is warmed.

A United Nations report stated that "it is too late to halt the effects from global warming, and nations should begin to prepare for rising sea levels and crop damage expected from the greenhouse effect."[10]

Bear in mind that climatic calamities such as heat waves, droughts, floods, and hurricanes can occur with ever-increasing frequency if the atmosphere only heats up by a mere 3 degrees to 8 degrees Fahrenheit.[11]

The Environmental Protection Agency (EPA) says that if present trends continue, the climate may change as much in the next 100 years as it has in the past 18,000 years . . . since the last ice age.[12]

THE PROBLEM IS REAL

Richard Somerville is the head of Scripps Institute of Oceanography's Climate Research Group, and stands at the forefront of international climatology. When asked if greenhouse warming has already changed our weather, he responded, "There's no disagreement in the scientific community: The greenhouse effect is a problem. We differ on the warming we expect, how quickly it will occur, and how it will be distributed over the Earth. But there's remarkable unanimity that it's a very, very real problem."[13]

Certainly we are witnessing some of the effects of these climatic changes now. We are seeing record heat levels at the equator and record cold temperatures at the poles. The fierce drought of 1988 was felt worldwide, especially in the United States and China.

Lester Brown, a noted agricultural economist and president of Worldwatch Institute, points out that the world output of grain has dropped for two consecutive years, with a percentage drop "larger than at any other time in history."[14]

A Department of Agriculture Report confirmed that 1988's winter wheat crop was the smallest in 11 years.[15] Kansas produced its worst yield in nearly a quarter century.[16] In the year 1988, the United States, perhaps for the first time in history, did not produce as much food as it consumed.[17] Floods in Bangladesh, hurricanes in Central America, and locusts in Africa were described by one U.N. official as "the most extensive in recorded history."[18]

The Worldwatch Institute estimates that disasters related to climate have already created some 10 million environmental refugees—people forced to evacuate areas where they cannot find enough food, potable water, or means of support.[19]

Most assuredly, the prospect of massive global warming is still open to much scientific debate, but the significance of these occurrences simply cannot be ignored now that the greenhouse effect has become so widely understood.

It is no wonder that people all over the world are troubled by this rapidly escalating problem. Over a decade ago, George F. Kennan, the distinguished U.S. diplomat, predicted that "environmental issues eventually would be as important as arms control on the national agenda."[20]

In early 1988, environmental ministers and other delegates from 124 nations met for an unprecedented conference to confront, as a group, the problems of a planet in distress and to discuss ways to spare the global environment from further destruction.

THE CHALLENGE IS UPON US

Of equal concern is the growing shortage of fresh water supplies and the increasing pollution of what we do have, as well as the availability of clean, breathable air.

As we step into the last decade before the 21st century, the health of our environment and the health of the planet that supports our lives is in the forefront of our consciousness. The environmental issue is, in fact, probably the most critical issue of our lifetime.

And this opinion is by no means shared only by those ecological groups who have long held that our environment requires more thought and attention.

The presidents of the National Academy of Sciences, National Academy of Engineering, and Institute of Medicine collectively made the statement: "We believe that global environmental change may well be the most pressing international issue of the next century."[21]

The annual economic summit in Paris in 1989, attended by the world's seven largest industrial democracies, ended with a formal communique that, for the first time ever, made the environment a top political priority.

The communique, which was 22 pages long, devoted a full 10 pages to the environment, compared to the previous year in which such issues barely received a paragraph. It warned of "an urgent need to safeguard the environment for future generations."[22]

ALL THINGS ARE CONNECTED

"And what," you may very well ask, "do animal products and heart attacks have to do with global warming and the greenhouse effect?

"What could atherosclerosis possibly have to do with carbon dioxide build-up and the weakening of the Earth's ecosystem?"

When most of us sit down to eat a meal, we haven't the slightest awareness of how our everyday food choices affect the health of our planet. But, in fact, all things are strongly connected. Everything is part of everything else. Nothing really stands alone. We don't always see the connection between one phenomenon and another, but the planet Earth is a living, breathing ecological entity held together by trillions of different occurrences that appear to be separate but are actually highly interconnected.

FOOD FOR THOUGHT

No one wants to leave his or her child the inheritance of a world that is uninhabitable. That fearful prospect may not seem to have anything to do with what you eat for dinner tonight, but it, in fact, has **everything** to do with it.

The great irony is that the industry producing the animal products we eat, those "foods" that clog our arteries and kill us—that same industry also contributes **enormously** to the pollution and suffocation of our planet. To say that the animal products industry is huge is like saying that the Grand Canyon is a big crack in the ground.

The production, feeding, growing, slaughtering, and transporting to market of **16 million animals every day**[23] for consumption is no small feat. The resources necessary to accomplish such a task are astronomical, and the resulting effect on the environment is devastating.

WASTE NOT—WANT NOT

It has been well established that, by far, the largest contributing factor to the assault on the environment is the reckless, runaway burning of fossil fuels, which accounts for 80 percent of the carbon dioxide in the atmosphere.[24]

We are all aware of the vast amounts of energy required to operate our automobiles, heat our homes, and produce the manufactured goods we buy. But few of us, indeed, understand what scope of energy is required to supply us with our meat-based diet. To describe it as colossal would be a gross understatement.

When I first uncovered this information, I had a difficult time adequately connecting fossil-fuel usage and the animal products industry, and I can understand if you are having that same difficulty now. Had I not delved deeply into this subject in particular, I might never have become aware of the staggering expenditure of our energy resources precipitated by the American appetite for animal products.

In fact, according to Dr. David Pimental of Cornell University, "If we use all of the known petroleum reserves strictly to produce food—no petroleum used for transportation, heating, cooling, and so forth—but just to produce food to feed the world population on our diet, using our agricultural technology, the world's known petroleum reserves would last a mere 12 years."[25]

And the food group that devours the lion's share of this energy for food production is made up of animal products—not fruits, vegetables, or any other food we may eat.

The protein we derive from beef takes at least 25 times more energy to produce than a comparable amount of protein from grain.[26] Animal agriculture is therefore responsible for 2,500 percent more consumption of fossil fuel than grain production.

We can measure our energy resources in terms of calories. In order to obtain only one calorie of protein from feedlot beef (the source of over 80 percent of the beef consumed in the U.S.),[27] an amazing 78 calories of fossil fuel has to be spent. Yet one calorie of protein from wheat, corn, or beans can be produced at the cost of only three-and-a-half calories of fossil fuel.[28]

THE ENERGY CONNECTION

Where is all this energy being used? When you drive down the highway behind a huge truck that is belching out thick plumes of black smoke, it's easy to make the connection between moving vehicles and energy usage. But ask people to make a connection between energy usage and sitting down to a breakfast of bacon and eggs, a hamburger for lunch, or a steak dinner, and they can't see the association.

SEVEN MORE DEADLY SINS . . .

As you will soon see, the chain of events that unfolds from the time an animal is born until it winds up on your dinner plate is one that appears to be designed specifically for the purpose of squandering our natural resources.

There are essentially seven areas of activity that account for the unexpectedly vast amounts of fossil fuel required to supply the industry that provides us with animal products. They are (1) production, (2) transportation, (3) processing, (4) storage, (5) packaging, (6) distribution, and (7) preparation.

Production. This is by far the most costly aspect of the animal products industry, in terms of energy expenditure. It encompasses everything that is done to or for the animals produced for food prior to their butchering.

Production includes the raising, housing, and feeding of the six billion animals earmarked for slaughter in this country every year. The agricultural aspects of supplying the food to feed such a mind-boggling number of animals is what accounts for the greatest expenditure of our nonrenewable energy in the area of production.

Can you even begin to imagine the amount of food it takes to feed **six billion animals?**

GORGING LIVESTOCK WHILE
PEOPLE GO HUNGRY

Most of the crops grown for food in this great, fertile country of ours are not even eaten by people—they're eaten by livestock destined for the slaughterhouse.

Tonight when you go to sleep, in towns all over the United States, there will be little girls and boys who will go to sleep hungry, wishing for some food to fill their empty stomachs. And as they dream of the food that won't be on the table the next morning, all over the country, livestock will be stuffed to the hilt on the very crops that **could** be feeding these children.

The most plentiful crop grown in America is corn. Of the total amount of corn that is eaten, almost 90 percent is consumed—not by human beings—but by livestock.[29]

Most of the oats, rye, barley, sorghum, and soybeans grown in this country are fed to livestock as well. In fact, in the United States, livestock consume five times as much grain as humans.[30] They eat enough grain and soybeans to feed over five times the entire human population of the country.[31] And yet . . . we have hungry children.

Of all vegetation produced by United States agriculture, 70 percent is consumed by livestock; 5 percent is consumed by the American people.[32]

(The remaining 25 percent is either exported, put aside for seed, or wasted in harvesting and/or processing.)

AMAZING . . . BUT TRUE

What truly stretches the imagination almost to the breaking point is when you try to fathom the amount of land it takes to grow all of that food. It is almost incomprehensible how much land is used to supply food and fodder for livestock.

The amount of land used to grow **all** food for human consumption in the United States is 60 million acres.[33]

The amount of land used to grow all of what is fed to livestock is over 1.2 **billion** acres.[34]

So, for every 60 acres of land used to grow food for people to eat, 1,200 acres are used to grow food for animals to eat.

That means that the land used to grow all food for human consumption is a mere **5 percent** of all land used to grow food. And what truly brings home most emphatically the extent of wastefulness associated with this statistic is the fact that Americans obtain a full two-thirds of their nutrition from this 5 percent of the land and only one-third of their nutrition from the 95 percent.[34A]

It requires over **500 times** as much land to produce a pound of beef than a pound of produce.[34B]

As startling as these numbers are, it's hard to grasp the full impact of the disparity between the two figures. To put it into a perspective that no one can miss, consider this: The 60 million acres used to grow food for human beings constitutes a land mass about the size of the state of Oregon.

STATING THE CASE

The 1.2 billion acres used to grow food for live-stock is equivalent to a land mass equal to the size of the states of Texas, California, Montana, New Mexico, Arizona, Nevada, Colorado, Wyoming, North Dakota, South Dakota, Pennsylvania, New York, North Carolina, South Carolina, Florida, Georgia, Illinois, Wisconsin, Indiana, Kentucky, Tennessee, Virginia, West Virginia, and Maine.

Over half of the land in this country is used to raise livestock! And it is the choicest half. The deserts and nonarable land are a good part of the remaining half. Discount Alaska, and it is **two- thirds!**

To merely state that the energy needed to grow and harvest this food is massive, seems, again, to be a gross understatement.

There are several areas of production that require energy:

A. The fleets of farm equipment, tractors, and farm trucks, in constant use, performing the day-to-day activities of running a farm. These vehicles, used to plow and till the soil, spread fertilizers, truck in food, haul away the prodigious amount of wastes, and perform other farm chores, are some of the least fuel-efficient vehicles and equipment in existence. They get perhaps a mile a gallon, or **less!**

B. Fertilizers are used extensively on these crops that are grown for food. Nitrogen, one of the main ingredients in fertilizer, is made by using natural gas. Twenty billion pounds of nitrogen is used a year.[35]

The natural gas used in the United States to make fertilizers is enough to fuel all of the gas-burning stoves, ovens, and other gas-burning appliances in the country.[36]

C. The water used to irrigate all of this land amounts to **trillions** of gallons. Imagine the energy required to supply the electricity to work the pumps that water this land.

D. Although this is neither the time nor the place to discuss the abominable horrors of factory farming, suffice it to say that today's factory farms are ghastly, austere places. Some of the structures in which animals are housed are so huge, that if you were to stand at one end of some of them, you could hardly see to the other side. Imagine a football field, enclosed, jam-packed with animals. These gigantic housing structures, and thousands of others of varying dimensions all over the country, have to be heated in cold weather and cooled when it is hot. The amount of energy needed to accomplish these tasks and all of the other activities requiring electricity and fuel is of massive proportions.

Transportation. Right at this moment, trucks and trains are criss-crossing this country with livestock animals. Cattle, for example, are transported from the farm to the feeding lot to the auction house, to the finishing lot, and then to the slaughterhouse. Once again, trucks and trains are some of the least fuel-efficient means of travel.

Processing. This is a polite word for the butchering or slaughtering of the six billion animals.

Highly mechanized slaughterhouses move animals through a sophisticated assembly line, using a tremendous amount of equipment, most of which runs off of electricity.

Also, the multibillion dollar dairy industry is almost entirely energy dependent. From the milking of cows to the processing of cheese and the pasteurizing of milk, an astronomical amount of equipment, all dependent on energy to operate, is necessary to run the gigantic dairy business in this country.

THE COLD, HARD FACTS

Storage. When talking about storage, think of refrigeration. From the time an animal is slaughtered until it finds its way onto the plate of the consumer, its flesh must be kept refrigerated. Why? Because the moment the animal is killed, it starts to decompose. Doesn't sound too appealing, but that's what happens. And the only ways to slow the process are with refrigeration or with chemicals such as sodium sulfite to reduce the smell of decay and keep the flesh pink. In which case, it will still have to be refrigerated.

Try to envision the refrigeration necessary to keep cold the various parts of six billion animals shipped and stored all over this country. Refrigeration requires a tremendous amount of energy. A great deal of this meat is also frozen, and freezing takes even more energy than refrigeration.

As a side note to this aspect of storage, the animal products industry is also contributing to the depletion of Earth's ozone layer.

Ozone molecules are destroyed by chlorofluoro-carbons (CFCs). One of the main sources of CFCs comes from **refrigerants**.

Packaging. After the carcasses have been sliced up, the various cuts are wrapped in individual packages for sale.

We're all familiar with these packages. The meat is placed on a styrofoam plate and covered in clear plastic wrap. Once again, an enormous amount of equipment is necessary to do the wrapping. By the way, the clear plastic wrap is a petroleum-based product. I don't know how much of this clear plastic wrap is used, but I wouldn't be surprised if it were enough to wrap the entire planet up a couple of thousand times. **Plus** . . . styrofoam produces CFCs, which are released into the atmosphere.

Distribution. Those gas-guzzling trucks and trains are put into use again. In this case, they are all equipped for either refrigeration or freezing. They are making their daily deliveries to literally hundreds of thousands of restaurants, grocery stores, and butcher shops, all of which are equipped with their own refrigeration to keep the meat cold or frozen.

WHAT'S COOKING

Preparation. We're now at the final step before consumption. And except for an occasional serving of steak tartare, meat is being cooked in restaurants and households all over this country. And that is one whole heck of a lot of stoves being fired up every day, which is one whole heck of a lot of energy being **burned** up.

All told, the energy requirements of the animal products industry represents a titanic, unrelenting drain on our country's energy resources.

After absorbing some of the facts from the last section (if you were not already aware of them), I would suspect that the next time you hear that someone is having difficulty connecting the consumption of a cheeseburger and a milkshake with the energy crisis in this country, you'll hardly know where to begin to explain.

It is exceedingly difficult to get a sense of the true magnitude of animal products' role in energy consumption. If you can, even for a moment, grasp the full extent of its impact, you could not help but be astounded—**and troubled.**

"A LITTLE BIT WON'T HURT . . ."
HOW ABOUT A TON?

Many of us are also deeply concerned about the ingestion of the pesticides that are sprayed on and added to our food, and most of us think that the greatest amount of these poisons are found on fruits and vegetables. However, that idea is just as erroneous as the notion that the sun is made of ice.

Of all the toxic chemical residues found in the food consumed by Americans, less than 10 percent comes from fruit, vegetables, and grains. **Over 90 percent comes from animal products.**[37] Factory farm animals have a dangerously high concentration of these chemical toxins in their bodies from a lifetime of eating feed that has been sprayed with these deadly biocides.

Many people who attend my health seminars invariably bombard me with fearful questions about what to do about all the pesticides on fruits and vegetables. Never—**not once**—has anyone raised the question of pesticides in meat, chicken, fish, eggs, or dairy products. Remarkable!

Animal products have **nine times** more pesticides, and **no one** seems to be aware of it. Getting stuck on the issue of pesticides in produce while eating animal products is a lot like worrying about getting your shoes wet in a puddle as a monstrous tidal wave is about to obliterate you.

In addition to the food we eat every day, there are two other essential elements without which we would quickly perish: water and air. Both surround us. Seventy percent of the surface of the earth is water; seventy percent of the human body is water.

We have a two-mile-thick layer of air around the earth weighing about six trillion tons. Without water we're dead in a matter of days—without air, in a matter of minutes. Few of us even have an inkling of the disastrous effect that the animal products industry has on these two precious resources.

JUST A COOL, CLEAR DRINK

First, let's talk about water. A great number of people became acutely aware of just how delicate the balance is between our water supply and our water needs after the disastrous drought of 1988. There is only a fixed amount of water available to us. A certain amount of it will be used, and a certain amount of what's left will be polluted.

The animal products industry uses more water than all other industries combined.[38] Mind you, it doesn't use more than any **other** industry; it uses more than **all** other industries **combined!** That is because the process of getting meat to your table is horribly inefficient and wasteful.

We have already learned the startling fact that only a small percentage of the acreage available for the harvesting of food in the United States is used to grow food for people. Practically all of the food grown is fed to livestock!

A nearly incomprehensible amount of water is necessary to grow all that food, only for it to be fed to livestock. As hard as this fact may be to accept, **over half of the water consumed in the United States is used in animal agriculture**, the greatest percentage of which goes to irrigate land growing feed for livestock.[39]

Try to envision vast fields farther than the eye can see, of alfalfa, soybeans, sorghum, oats, and other grains being saturated with millions of jet-streams of water.

WATER, WATER, EVERYWHERE?

Enough water goes into the production of **one** steer to float a U.S. naval destroyer![40]

The growing of one pound of wheat requires only 25 gallons of water, while the production of one pound of meat requires two-and-a-half **thousand** gallons![41]

In fact, so much water is used by the animal products industry that it has to be subsidized by the government, with **your** tax dollars. If this were not the case, the least expensive cut of beef at your market would cost $35 a pound, just as it does in Japan, where the water is **not** subsidized. We are talking about hundreds of billions of dollars. (In California **alone**, the cost of subsidizing the meat industry is $24 billion a year!)

This subsidized water winds up being so absurdly inexpensive to the industry that it is 2,000 times less expensive than sand![42]

Perhaps you are familiar with the Ogallala Aquifer. This is an almost incomprehensibly huge body of water that flows underneath the Western Great Plains.

Fifty years ago it was considered to be a virtually inexhaustible reservoir of water. But we have been tapping into the Aquifer with increasing regularity, to the point where over 35 billion gallons a day are withdrawn—over 13 trillion gallons a year![43]

Now it is estimated that the great Ogallala Aquifer will be dry in 35 to 40 years, leaving the Great Plains of the United States uninhabitable.[44] The vast majority of the water being removed, which is threatening this wonder of nature, is, of course, being used to produce meat.

Even the mighty Colorado River, the carver of the Grand Canyon, which has been gushing headlong into the open sea for ages, is no longer what it once was. The water of the Colorado is used up before it can even reach the ocean. Once again, the greatest amount goes to produce meat.

And what about the water that's left? The animal products industry is responsible for the pollution of more water than all other industries combined![45]

Once again, not more than any **other** industry, but more than **all** other industries **combined!**

WHAT A PILE . . .

One major cause of this devastating pollution is the fact that **every second**, 250,000 pounds of excrement are produced by livestock in this country.[46] That is over seven and a half trillion pounds of animal excrement a year, for which there is no sewage system.

Therefore, every year, most of this animal excrement finds its way into our water. Believe it or not, the U.S. Department of Agriculture used to have a policy of encouraging beef producers to situate feedlots on hillsides near streams in order to facilitate the easy channeling of waste into the water.[47]

The other **major** source, in fact, the **primary** source of water pollution in the United States, is from erosion of agricultural land, the vast majority of which is used to produce animal products. The runoff from these lands carries an immense quantity of deadly biocides (fungicides, herbicides, pesticides, etc.), inorganic minerals, and soil particles into our waterways, all of which contribute to the animal products industry's pollution of more water than all other human activities combined.

WE ARE WHAT WE DRINK

In 1989 both a Gallup poll and a Louis Harris poll showed that an overwhelming number of Americans (over 70 percent) are deeply concerned about water pollution issues. In both polls the **number one** concern, over dumping of toxic wastes, air pollution, deforestation, loss of agricultural land, acid rain, and pesticide use, was water quality.[48]

That being the case, the fact that the industry supplying us with animal products is not only **using** more water than all other industries combined but is also **polluting** more of what's left, is a situation screaming out to be rectified.

Perhaps these appalling facts about our water supply would be more palatable if, at the very least, all this food, land, and water was used in the most efficient manner possible. But the process of cycling our food through livestock is ridiculously inefficient **and** wasteful.

It takes 30 pounds of vegetation to produce only one pound of beef.[49] As a result, we lose 90 percent of its protein value and 100 percent of its fiber and carbohydrates.[50] Plus, the same acre of land that will produce only 165 pounds of beef will yield **20,000 pounds** of potatoes.[51]

And all of this waste occurs so that we might be supplied with a product that has been medically proven to be a leading contributor to the number-one cause of death in this country.

THAT'S NOT ALL, FOLKS

If we were to stop here, there would be more than sufficient reason to seriously consider reducing our dependency on a meat-based diet. Taking into account the number of deaths from heart disease and stroke, the pitifully inefficient and wasteful use of our land and food, and the squandering and pollution of our water, we have more than ample cause to rethink our priorities. However, even this is not the full picture—not by a long shot.

THE BREATH OF LIFE

Let's consider the one necessity of life we can least afford to do without: air. Air is our most urgent need, crucial to our existence under **all** conditions. We can go for months without food, for days without water, but six minutes without air, and we're dead. In your lifetime, you will consume more weight in air than in food and water **combined**.

However, no discussion of air can be complete without talking about . . . **TREES!** Why? Because as part of the splendor, intelligence, and magnificence of Mother Nature, trees contribute to the grand system of symbiosis between the plant and animal kingdoms.

When you behold the exquisite nature of our interrelationship with trees, you can't help but stand in awe of the remarkable wisdom that underlies the connectedness of all living things.

When we breathe in a lungful of life-giving air, our bodies extract the oxygen needed, and with every exhalation, they release carbon dioxide. Trees take up the carbon dioxide, use it in their own life processes, and give off oxygen. What an arrangement!

IS IT GETTING STUFFY IN HERE?

Carbon dioxide can be deadly. Breathing air that is only 3 percent carbon dioxide will make you noticeably drowsy. Concentrations any larger than that will usher you to your grave. Every 24 hours, the amount of carbon dioxide eliminated from your lungs is equal to a lump of charcoal weighing eight ounces.[52]

The oxygen/carbon dioxide balance on our planet is **not** something we can afford to mess around with. If carbon dioxide levels should **increase** massively while there is a corresponding **decrease** in oxygen, it doesn't take too much figuring to realize that we could ultimately be faced with a shortage of oxygen in the air.

The subject of the carbon dioxide and oxygen balance cannot be excluded from any discussion of the present global warming/greenhouse effect.

As we become more and more insistent that this life-threatening dilemma be dealt with **now**, before it is too late to do anything about it, the obvious questions are: "What is causing this situation?" and "How can we stop it?"

Fully one-half of the problem is due to the staggering increase in the amount of carbon dioxide that has been released into the atmosphere in recent decades. As stated earlier, this acceleration stems from the vast supplies of fossil fuels we burn . . . and it has caught up with us. Burning fossil fuels is the number-one source of the increase in carbon dioxide levels worldwide.

NOT THE TREES—PLEASE!

Naturally, our friends, the trees, through the process of photosynthesis, can and will put a huge dent in that carbon dioxide level. But here's the irony! At a time when carbon dioxide levels are becoming dangerously high, to the point of damaging the very environment in which we live, instead of expending every effort to protect and even increase the existing number of trees to counteract this madness, **we are instead decimating our forests at a frightening pace!**

These forests are our planet's most important air purifiers, so this destruction defies all reason! It's like trying to put out a fire by throwing kerosene on it. Forests all over the world are being cut, burned, and cleared at the stupefying rate of **40 million acres a year!**[53]

That is over **100,000 acres every single day! More than one acre per second!***

---

*There are estimates, from knowledgeable sources, who place the number at **twice** this amount.

The United States has already lost an estimated 260 million acres of highly productive forestland to agriculture.[54] That leaves less than 200 million acres of this highly productive forestland, and much of it is understocked. If you fly over Oregon and Washington, you can see vast patches of skinned earth where every remnant of forest has been removed.

Going by the rate at which U.S. forests were cleared between 1967 and 1977—the latest period for which there is reliable data—all forests in the United States will be stripped bare in 50 years' time!

What is so ironic and frustrating is that this on-going catastrophe could be turned around. Robin Hur, Harvard Business School graduate and author, has been researching and studying these matters for over a quarter of a century, is of the opinion that of the 260 million acres of prime U.S. forestland that has already been cut down for agricultural purposes, 200 million acres could be transformed back into highly productive land by raising food to feed people instead of livestock.[55]

The pervasive policy of **increasing** carbon dioxide levels while **decreasing** oxygen-producing and carbon dioxide-consuming forests borders on planetary suicide.

The great irony is that deforestation itself accounts for 20 percent of the increase in carbon dioxide levels.[56] So, when trees are cut, not only do we lose their carbon dioxide-consuming capabilities, but we are also hit with an increase in carbon dioxide as they are destroyed. No wonder our environment is exhibiting such stress. It is sounding an alarm, crying out for help!

TRADING TREES FOR HAMBURGERS

"What do animal products have to do with forests?" you may ask. Well, the astonishing answer is: **The vast majority of the forestland that is cleared is used for grazing livestock or for growing livestock feed!** We're deforesting the heartland of our country and the world to supply Americans with animal products, which we consume by the ton, so we can die from heart attacks.

In the United States, for every acre of trees cleared to make room for parking lots, roads, houses, shopping centers, etc., **seven acres** are destroyed to grow feed for livestock or to graze cattle.[57]

All over the world, North America, Central America, South America, the Amazon, Asia, Africa, Australia—wherever trees grow—they are being cut away, mostly for the purpose of raising livestock—a good percentage of which goes to the United States **to be sold as fast-food hamburgers!**

OUR PRECIOUS RAINFORESTS

The tropical rainforests of the world are probably Earth's most precious natural resource, offering refuge to three-quarters of all living things on the planet.[58] Of the 25 percent of the surface of Earth that is not covered by water, fully one-third is blanketed by a lush green belt of forest frequently referred to as "Earth's lungs"—appropriately named when you consider that trees are such a critical link in Earth's neverending effort to maintain a proper oxygen/carbon dioxide balance.

These lush, emerald havens of life support a nearly unbroken canopy of 200-foot trees as far as the eye can see, and they are virtually teeming with a symphony of insects, birds, monkeys, and other living creatures. The abundance of flowering plants and other vegetation in the rain forests is of such beauty and diversity as to take your breath away. Some species of plants found there have never been seen outside a rainforest. Yet, these tropical forests are being wiped out at the rate of 27 million acres a year![59]

One hundred years ago, when automobiles were a new invention and airplanes were only a dream, the tropical rainforests were a mysterious, challenging unknown. Today the challenge is to prevent them from disappearing. One-half of the world's tropical rainforests, which were standing at the beginning of this century, have now been destroyed.

Dr. Paul Ehrlich, Professor of Biological Science at Stanford University, speaking on rainforest destruction, stated, "Second only to nuclear war, there are few problems more critical to humanity at the moment."[60]

When Isaac Asimov was asked by Bill Moyers on a news interview what he considered to be the most urgent problems addressed by society, he said, "Population and the rainforest."[61]

To illustrate what is happening to the rainforests, let's look at Central America. Presently, 260 acres of forest are destroyed every day to produce grazing area for beef cattle.[62] This statistic not only reflects local consumption, but also the **90 percent** exported to the United States.[63] This type of destruction is taking place in all of the tropical rainforests of the world!

WHEN IS ENOUGH ENOUGH?

Our country's appetite for meat-based products almost seems insatiable. Although 75 percent of the children under five years of age in Guatemala are undernourished, that country uses its land and food resources to raise cattle to export 40 million pounds of meat to the United States every year.[64] I'm sure you would agree: That's not just wrong, that's wrong to the nth degree.

In total, the United States imports 138 million pounds of beef from Central America annually.[65] Many people feel outraged by this kind of gluttony. Here we are, already slaughtering six billion animals a year, and still **that's not enough!** There are also many other countries who are using their resources to raise cattle to send millions and millions **more** pounds of beef to us while **their own children go hungry.**

In 1980, when the United States first began to import its beef, Central America boasted of 130,000 square miles of lush rainforests. Now, fewer than 80,000 square miles remain.[66] Recently, many public figures and celebrities have taken up the cause to save the rainforests of Brazil. One, in particular, the rock star Sting, undertook a multicountry tour with Raoni, a Brazilian Indian chieftain, as part of the campaign to reduce the destruction of the rainforests and to create a nature reserve in the Amazon River basin.

The Amazon, once one of the most prodigious expanses of rainforest in the world, has already been reduced by the destruction of nearly 100 million acres.[67] **Almost 75 percent of that loss is due to cattle ranching!**[68]

Surprisingly, cattle ranching in Amazonia is not even economical. Without heavy government subsidies and tax credits, almost all ranches would fail.[69] How ironic that the Brazilian government is actually paying to have its rainforests destroyed.

Susan Meeker-Lowry, author of "Economics As If the Earth Really Mattered," states: "It is essential that we understand the **extreme urgency** of the situation we face. If the destruction continues at its present rate, the tropical rainforests will be totally gone in 30 years."[70]

THE WAY OF THE DINOSAURS?

If even one species of **anything** were to be found on the moon or on one of the other planets in our solar system, it would be the most momentous event in history. Yet the destruction of tropical rainforests to clear grazing land for cattle is causing the mass extinction of 17,500 species of animals and plants a year.[71] Nearly 50 every day! Peter Raven of the Missouri Botanical Garden predicts that that number will double over the next three decades.[72]

We are pushing our earthly companions toward extinction at least a thousand times faster than at any other time in history.[73] Eating animal products not only predisposes you to an atherosclerotic death, but also helps to rob the planet of one of its greatest treasures.

BILLIONS AND BILLIONS DESTROYED

Eating hamburgers and hot dogs in our country is practically a national pastime. In fact, these foods are known worldwide as inherently "American," and we certainly support that idea, as we consume them by the millions of tons. Hamburgers and hot dogs are sold on thousands of street corners throughout our country. Their all-too-familiar advertisements and billboards relentlessly entice us to buy more. What is less familiar and certainly not as enticing is what this national pastime is costing our environment.

For every quarter pound of beef you eat from a steer raised in Central America, 55 square feet of rainforest had to be destroyed.[74]

The clearing of that much land contributes 500 pounds of carbon dioxide to the atmosphere.[75] That sheds a different light on the nonchalant American habit of picking up a burger and fries whenever the impulse strikes, doesn't it?

Unfortunately, the scope of global problems obscures the fact that they are the result of billions of individual actions. It's difficult for each of us to see how our personal activities influence the overall situation. When we try to tackle a problem as huge as the threat to our environment, it is nearly impossible to measure the effect of one person's effort to improve the condition. Well, here is a way to **know** that your actions are not lost among the statistics:

If, over a year's time, you have one less hamburger a week, you could potentially be saving over two-and-a-half thousand square feet of rainforest, while preventing an additional 26,000 pounds of carbon dioxide from being spewed into our atmosphere.

In the words of Florentin Krause, the chairman of the International Project for Sustainable Energy Paths, "If we're losing forests in the Third World, we have to add it here. The only way to do it is to reduce beef and dairy consumption."[75A]

Of course, the United States is not the only country playing a part in the destruction of the world's rainforests. Due to its immense need for raw materials, Japan, too, has assumed a major role in world deforestation.

Twenty-five percent of all timber logged in the United States is shipped to Japan.[76] **Eighty percent** of the oldest living trees in the world from the Sarawak rainforests of Malaysia are shipped to Japan as well, for the manufacture of throwaway chopsticks (over 11 billion pair a year)[77] and plywood sheets, used two or three times for molding concrete and then **discarded.**[78]

In addition, the Japanese government is negotiating to build a $300 million, 500-mile road through the Amazon and over the Andes to the Peruvian coast, in order to acquire **more** trees, more quickly.[79]

According to the Worldwide Fund for Nature, "Japan's use of tropical rainforests is the most environmentally damaging in the world."[80]

A TREASURE TROVE

Few of us are aware that **trees are a renewable source of energy.** The fact that trees can supply energy, just like oil, gas, or coal, is practically ignored in our country. The six resources from which we obtain energy in the United States are:

Oil	–	38.5%
Gas	–	25.5%
Coal	–	23.0%
Nuclear Power	–	6.4%
Hydro Power	–	3.8%
Wood	–	2.5%

As you can see, at present, wood plays an almost insignificant role in our energy supply. Of all the energy resources listed above, coal is, without question, the dirtiest. (Solar energy, not yet in use enough to be listed above, is the cleanest.) When we burn coal, there is no way to ignore the filth that it creates in our environment. As we take the necessary steps to discontinue harmful (and avoidable) practices, a reduction in the use of coal is a good place to start.

Over the past 20 years, research has been ongoing in Wisconsin to develop a system of growing trees, harvesting them to fuel wood-burning electric power plants, and then immediately regrowing the trees. Trees 60 to 70 feet tall can be grown in 8 to 12 years, harvested, used for fuel, and regrown. The tree farms producing this natural fuel are called Short-Rotation Energy Plantations.[81]

If we would continue to refine the technology, wood could replace coal altogether. The trees would not create the filth in the environment that coal produces, and while they were growing, they would also produce oxygen and reduce carbon dioxide in the atmosphere.

Tree farms also have other advantages over coal mining. They prevent the strip-mining that coal requires. If you have ever seen land after it has been strip-mined for coal, you know that it is a grotesque blight against Nature that can only be likened in ugliness to the effects of a nuclear holocaust.

Tree farms also generate more money than the same acreage of land, cleared for grazing. A recent study indicates that a tree plantation on a hectare of land (2½ acres) can net $3,184, compared to pastureland, which yields only $2,960.[82]

One recent study in the British journal, *Nature*, pointed out that the products yielded by the Amazonian rainforest (rubber, produce, etc.) could generate **more than TWICE the income of either cattle ranching or lumbering.**[83]

Cultural Survival, a Cambridge, Massachusetts organization, has plans to import $50 million a year in rainforest products such as oils, resins, honey, pigments, and fibers.[84]

The more we investigate the role of trees on our planet, the more we understand just how valuable they are.

MOTHER EARTH

While I am on the subject of resources we treasure, what would you guess is the most valuable of Earth's resources? What is more precious than diamonds or gold?

SOIL.

Now, before you dismiss what I am saying as nonsensical, consider this: If there was ever a food shortage, you couldn't eat priceless gems, but you **could** grow food provided you had good soil.

Archeological and historical research based on scientific analysis of soil, vegetation, and landscape evolution indicates that the fall of many great civilizations, including Egypt, Greece, and Rome, was due in part to ecological considerations.[85] In the final stages before collapse, devastating military struggles were fought—not for wealth or ideology—but for the control of arable land and essential resources.

Soil erosion is the most serious threat to our planet at present. Without soil, the terrain of planet Earth would be as lifeless as the moon.

SOIL IS NOT DIRT!

In fact, in the farm areas of this country, I have seen bumper stickers that say: "Please Don't Treat Our Soil Like Dirt." Great advice. Topsoil is actually the dark, nutrient-rich soil that supplies us with our nutritional requirements by feeding the plants that we eat.

Two hundred years ago cropland had, on the average, about 21 inches of topsoil in which to grow our food. Today, that number has dropped to six inches.[86] We lose another inch every 20 years.[87]

The United States Soil Conservation Service states that four million acres of agricultural land are lost due to erosion every year.[88] There is an annual loss of our precious topsoil of **six billion tons**, which is 50,000 pounds for every man, woman, and child in our country.

Worldwide, the total loss is 25 billion tons a year.[89] What makes these statistics more ominous is the fact that it takes Nature an average of 350 years to build just **one inch** of topsoil.[90]

The major factor involved in this truly tragic loss of life-sustaining topsoil is the raising of livestock.

Eighty-five percent of our topsoil loss is directly associated with livestock production.[91] This astonishing fact ought to motivate us to begin making new food choices. The only factor preventing the starvation of us and our children is the **soil**. Clearing the land for livestock grazing causes it to be blown away in the wind and washed away in our rivers. Once it's gone, it's gone.

The present rate of loss simply must be halted. **We need the soil to grow our food!** It is simply too precious a resource to be treated with such unconscious disdain.

On the other hand, ungrazed forests are one of the only places where the erosion of topsoil is not a problem. It's only after the forests are cleared or when cattle are allowed to graze among the trees that the rapid loss of topsoil begins.

Why? Trees are the planet's chief means for building and protecting topsoil for several reasons. First, their roots create new soil and supply existing soil with a constant source of mineral nutrients by breaking down and dissolving bedrock. Secondly, the roots of trees keep the soil moisturized by drawing up deep groundwater. Thirdly, roots help bind the soil, protecting it from wind and water erosion. Lastly, the foliage of trees protects soil from the sun. Without tree cover, forestland turns to desert.

You may be surprised to learn that most of the world's deserts were formerly forests or woodlands, **including the Sahara**, which was stripped of its trees by the Roman Empire to make way for vast grainfields.

Upwards of 150 million acres of United States forestland is available for grazing by cattle.[92]

HOME, HOME ON THE DESERT

The word "desertification" was coined by a French scientist in the 1940s. The term is used to describe arid yet **productive** land that has been impoverished and despoiled, either by nature or by human activity. The silting up of scarce rivers and streams, the accumulation of salt in the soil (salinization), and excessive soil erosion are the symptoms of land being turned into desert.

One tends to think of Africa when thinking of good land that has been "desertified." We've all seen pictures of scorched, dry, cracked land without a blade of grass for miles. We've also seen the starving millions who can no longer grow food for themselves on such barren, forsaken land.

The United Nations Environmental Program reports that 15 million acres in arid regions are turned into unreclaimable desert every year and that another 50 million acres a year are placed at risk.[93]

But not here in the United States!

I wish I could say that were true.

In 1976, researchers at a United Nations conference on this subject in Nairobi, Kenya, reported that
the United States was undergoing severe desertification, which in places, was **worse** than Africa's.[94]
Those warnings were ignored. In the last decade, as
is true with other problems that are disregarded, the
situation did not go away; it became worse.

Millions of acres in the western half of the United
States are being affected by the phenomenon of
desertification. The Council on Environmental Quality has confirmed this with a report that included a
map of the West's desertification, drawn by Harold
Dregne, one of the nation's leading experts on this
subject. It showed that 36.8 percent of the North
American continent's dry land has suffered "severe"
desertification.

We are talking about the great, vast, beautiful rangeland of the West, which was the inspiration for "Home, home on the range, where the deer and the antelope play." Well, they are not playing there any longer. What is the cause of this national tragedy?

Considering some of the revelations in this book so far, it should be no surprise to you that, once again, our meat habit forces us to take direct responsibility for this blight against our land. In the words of Richard Rice, a resource economist with the Wilderness Society, "Cattle are the scourge of the Earth."[95]

The world-renowned conservationist, John Muir, referred to cattle as "hooved locusts."[96] This is a unique, but environmentally relevant way for all of us to regard them.

The Council on Environmental Quality states that "overgrazing, as it has come to be known, has been the most potent desertification force, in terms of total acreage affected, within the United States."[97]

Jim Mower, staff officer for range and wildlife on the Wasatch-Cache National Forest in Utah, says that many ranges he inspected last summer ". . . are so overgrazed, there isn't enough fuel on the ground to start a fire."[98] It's what author Edward Abbey referred to when he called the Rocky Mountain West "cowburnt."

Scientists have pointed out for years that cattle grazing has destroyed more Western land than all other human activities combined.[99]

The General Accounting Office in June of 1988 noted that the number of cattle on public land still exceeds the land's carrying capacity.[100]

WHOSE LAND IS IT ANYWAY?

This is **our** land! Federally run **public** land. Land that was supposed to be **preserved** for the **perpetual pleasure and use** of **all** Americans. Yet somehow the cattle ranchers have obtained the right to do whatever they want to this public land. How can this be if the land belongs to us? The United States Forest Service, an arm of the United States Department of Agriculture, whose **sole** function is to promote the interests of farmers and ranchers, and the Bureau of Land Management, known derisively as the "Bureau of Livestock Management," have **leased** the land to the cattle ranchers!

Over 170 million acres of **our** land has been leased. If the ranchers want to cut every tree, saturate the land with pesticides and herbicides, ravage the ground so severely that riverbanks collapse, making the water so thick with mud that trout suffocate as they try to spawn, then they can. They can make our irreplaceable biological heritage, this wide open rangeland, unfit for anything.

And what price would you imagine is being paid for the right to do this to our land? On the average, an astonishing **3.2¢ per acre per month!**[101]

After fending off critics for years who expressed indignation at the scandalously low fees, the Bureau of Land Management finally, in 1989, raised the monthly grazing fees to almost **4¢ per acre.** The cost to the federal agencies to just administer the grazing program is three times that amount. If you are suspicious about where the shortfall of approximately $30 to $50 million comes from, your suspicions are justified. It **does** come from your wallet. This destructive use of public land is subsidized by your tax dollars.

Understandably, the legitimate question in many minds is: "How on earth could an agency (Bureau of Land Management) set up within our government ostensibly to protect public land for the people who **are** the public, be so manipulated in favor of a private interest group?"

From 1979 to 1988, when so much of the abuse of this land occurred, the head of the Bureau of Land Management (appointed by President Reagan) was **a Colorado cattle rancher!**[102]

HERE TODAY, GONE TOMORROW

It seems that because we live in the "land of plenty," there is an attitude that there will **always** be plenty. We are rapidly finding out that our natural resources are finite, and without judicious use of these resources, we can exhaust them.

I must apologize. I have tried my best to maintain an air of objectivity while imparting the data in this book. But when I reflect on the fact that our craving for meat and other animal products is contributing greatly to the slow and inexorable destruction of everything of real value in this country—**with the help of our tax dollars**—I can't hide my feelings.

Our appetite for animal products is wiping out our trees, fouling our water, polluting our air, gobbling up our natural resources, and decimating our land. The unbearable irony is that these activities are for the purpose of supplying products that are also **killing our people!** I'm sorry, but I cannot mask my sadness with niceties.

LET'S TURN THE CORNER

Considering everything that you have read thus far, it would not be surprising for you to be losing faith in our country, from an environmental standpoint. However, it is important that you be aware of exactly what is going on.

But the negative side is only **part** of this incredible, but true, saga. There is, of course, another side of the story of equal or greater importance, as you will see when you turn the page.

PART II

The Solution

NO! IT'S NOT TOO LATE

And now, dear reader, here's the good news.

Perhaps the preceding pages have given you the feeling that there **is** no good news, that we are dealing with a lost cause, with problems so big and so runaway that they are insurmountable. Perhaps you are rightfully feeling that your life is already complicated and demanding enough, that mortgage and car payments are just about as much as you can handle without taking on the greenhouse effect and all of its contributing factors. In all likelihood, you want to help, but honestly feel overwhelmed by the magnitude of the problem.

But perhaps you don't realize the impact that **one person** can have on such a global dilemma.

That's what the second half of this book is about, and precisely because there are so many of us who **do** have a genuine willingness to make a difference, I feel confident that the information that follows **can** help to turn this seemingly hopeless situation around. The truth is, our willingness is our saving grace.

It is well known that we have not yet passed the point of no return. All we need to do is see to it that changes are made. Gilbert M. Grosvenor, president and chairman of the board of the National Geographic Society, points out that "large-scale efforts around the world have shown that soil erosion and desertification can be arrested when the proper effort is made. Tropical forests do not have to be leveled to feed people."[103]

In a most valuable and informative book entitled, *Blueprint for a Green Planet*, the authors, John Seymour and Herbert Girardet, who have been involved in ecological studies for over half a century, present a most positive and encouraging formula for change. In their words, "There **are** things that the ordinary person can do. The world's decline is not inevitable. We are **not** powerless. We **can** prevent the deluge. If each of us—each individual—simply becomes aware of the dangers and does what he or she can do to avoid them, then as a species, we can continue to inhabit this planet. Far from turning our world into a wasteland, we can turn it into a paradise again."

Helping us in the quest to reverse the trend are two very positive factors favoring the success of the endeavor. First, the planet, being a living organism, is predisposed to healing itself. If you cut your finger, without any action on your part, your body will heal the wound. Healing will always occur, **unless** the wound is continually abused and reopened.

The planet has the same capacity. It will heal itself, **IF . . . the proper environment for healing is supplied.**

If we will only stop destroying it, it will not remain as it is; it will regenerate itself.

Secondly, the solution is so profoundly simple, so do-able and effective, that positive results can be realized in a very short period of time, with no drain on your personal time or energy.

YOU ARE THE MOST IMPORTANT FACTOR

What is most encouraging is that this is an **individual** solution. It does not have to appeal to government bureaucracies that can't seem to act before commissions meet to form committees, which, in turn, try to gain support and funding. It isn't threatened by the mountains of red tape that all too frequently choke even the most worthy and urgent projects before they can get off the ground. Nor does it rely on painstaking efforts to achieve some measure of industry reform.

This solution, in the truest sense, is "in the hands of the people."

Each and every person willing to help **can** make a difference. No one person has any more or less significance than any other. The more who participate, the more far-reaching and impactful will be the results. We will all have the opportunity to get involved, to belie the sentiments in Mark Twain's statement that "everybody complains about the weather, but nobody does anything about it." Although the problems seem to go far beyond the scope of one person, and regardless of what others may say or do, **your voice will be heard!**

THE TEN-PERCENT SOLUTION

The solution requires no training, no committees, no meetings, no marching in the streets, no letter-writing campaigns, no legislative efforts. It costs **nothing**. In fact, it will save you money. It is simple and effective, and here's how it works:

We all make a commitment to
***one vegetarian day* a week.**

That's it, one day a week you simply eat no meat, chicken, fish, eggs, or dairy products. That doesn't mean that on that day you go hungry. Not at all! On that day, you can have plenty to eat . . .

You can eat fruit, fruit salads and juices, nuts, vegetable dishes, salads of all kinds, pastas, soups, breads, rice and other grains, potatoes, lentils, beans, and other legumes.

No, there is no need to go hungry.

Using the **Ten Percent Solution**, all you are doing is eating 10 percent less food derived from animals and 10 percent more food derived from plants.

THAT'S IT?

At first, you may ask, "One vegetarian day a week? What is that going to do, considering the enormity of what has to be accomplished?" It's not difficult for one person to commit to one day, is it?

However, when millions of people all over the country make that commitment, and their efforts are viewed collectively, can you begin to see the potential in this collective effort?

THE FRUITS OF YOUR LABOR

If the consumption of animal products were decreased in the United States by a **mere 10 percent**, the ramifications would be astounding.

ONE

On a personal level, you will significantly reduce your chances of developing atherosclerosis, thereby lowering your risk of suffering from heart disease or stroke.

If you have children and they participate in one vegetarian day a week, you lay the foundation for a healthy heart for them now, and also later in their lives, while educating them early about dietary prudence and the measure of control they can have over their health.

TWO

Over one and a half trillion gallons of pure water will be saved a year.[104] That is equivalent to over three million gallons of precious water being saved every minute of every hour of every day of the year.

THREE

Nearly a half a trillion pounds of animal excrement a year will **not** be dumped into our waterways.[105]

FOUR

The reduced need for fuel will lower fossil fuel demands by the equivalent of 2.3 billion gallons a year.[106] That's a saving of over six million gallons a **day.**

FIVE

Every year we will have the benefit of the oxygen output and carbon dioxide consumption of 25 million acres of trees that would not otherwise exist.[107]

SIX

Twelve million tons of grain will be freed up a year.[108] That is more than enough grain to feed every one of the 20 million people who die of starvation and related diseases in the world every year.[109]

(That is one death from starvation **every one and a half seconds** without stop.)

There are those who would say that even if the food were freed up and made available, somehow it would still have to be brought to the people. True. But at least they would have a chance of receiving it. There is **no** chance if it's all fed to livestock.

SEVEN

Seven hundred million tons of topsoil will be saved a year.[110]

EIGHT

One hundred and twenty million acres of land, choice land, would be made available for more prudent use.[111]

NINE

Six hundred million animals a year will be saved from the slaughterhouse.[112]

LET THE HEALING BEGIN

Our environment will start to heal itself, because we will have taken major steps to provide the conditions for healing. There will be less pollution, more water, cleaner water, more air, cleaner air, less suffering, less death, **more life**.

All this from one vegetarian day a week. With such impressive changes coming from only one vegetarian day a week, can you imagine the repercussions from two vegetarian days a week? That would be an equivalent of more than a 25 percent reduction in animal product consumption and a more than **doubling** of the positive results listed above. Dare we dream?

The magnitude of the beneficial results that will occur from this one simple activity certainly shows us how much power we have in bringing about change.

The understanding of the impact that our food choices have on our environment is a new awareness for most people—so new, in fact, that even many **environmentalists** are oblivious of the connection. There are those who have dedicated their lives to the correct stewardship of the planet who still eat animal products three times a day every day without understanding the profound benefits that would result—in addition to everything else they are doing—if they would only slightly alter their choice of foods.

Up until now, this information has not been readily available to us. What is most important, of course, is what we will do once we **have** the information.

IT'S NOW OR NEVER

We have a totally unique opportunity. Never before in the history of this planet have the problems with the environment that we are presently confronting been so great an issue for such large numbers of people.

If **we** don't do what is necessary to turn things around, no future generation will have to deal with them either. Because there will not be anything to deal with. It will all have been lost.

Lester Brown, president of the Washington-based Worldwatch Institute, states, "We do not have generations, we only have years."[113]

CAN YOU TURN YOUR BACK?

As an inhabitant of planet Earth, is doing nothing even an option? After learning how simple and how small your effort would be, and understanding the profound changes that it would bring about in relation to your own personal health **and** to the health of our environment, can you even consider the possibility of doing nothing?

To paraphrase the words of Edmund Burke, "No greater mistake could be made in life than doing nothing because you could only do a little."

When a lot of people do a little, it's a **lot**. When a lot of people do nothing—it's **nothing**.

THE CHALLENGE IS UPON US

Our food choices DO make a difference! It is an affront and an insult to our intelligence and a threat to our survival to allow the situation to continue unchecked, as if the link were **not** there or **not** known. If the trend is not **at least** altered, where will it end?

To paraphrase an old saying, "If we're not careful, we're going to wind up where we're headed." The assault on our health and on our environment resulting from our reliance on a meat-based diet could conceivably have been the inspiration for that saying.

WHERE WERE YOU
DURING THE WAR, DADDY?

When the time comes for us to hand over the reins of the planet to our children, at the very least, it ought to be in as good a shape as when we took command—or even better. Certainly not worse!

We are all being faced with the challenge to be real-life heroes. Not figuratively speaking, but in all actuality. Future generations are going to look back at this time in history. They will see that in the 1990s we had the opportunity to ignore the problem, allowing it to reach disastrous irreversibility, or to step forward, with strength and courage, to rise above the apathy by doing our part. Will our children and grandchildren be able to look back with gratitude and praise for our foresight and action, or will they be forced to look back in bewilderment and anger at what we had, but destroyed, and allowed to be lost forever?

There is nothing that can break through the power of millions of people joined together with a common resolve to achieve a common goal. The tremendous benefits we can achieve by a 10 percent reduction in animal-product consumption, with one vegetarian day a week, are **real** and will absolutely come to pass.

This is not pie-in-the-sky! It's not wishful thinking! This is a **very achievable goal**. And all of those with vested interests, who would like to see things remain just as they are, will have to come around in their thinking. All we have to do is **DO IT!**

WE ARE IN THE DRIVER'S SEAT

Just remember that the less we consume of a product, the less of it will have to be produced. In this case, as we reduce the production of animal products, we lessen the resulting destruction to our environment to the same degree. Period!

Nothing changes that equation. It's the law of supply and demand. The sole factor determining the extent to which the environment will continue to be imperiled by our reliance on animal products is totally up to you, me . . . **US!**

It would be so easy to point a finger at the animal products industry and lay the blame on their doorstep. But the truth is, they are merely carrying out our bidding.

The animal products industry has no power whatsoever in this matter. If we demand that they produce more, they will; and if we demand that they produce less, they will. So, you and I are holding a most awesome responsibility in the palms of our hands. We alone can rescue the environment from this threat to its survival. Merely make a **slight** decrease in your own consumption of animal products . . . and arouse the awareness in others of the good, both individually and globally, that this activity will create. We can then be well on our way to turning this situation around.

Mostafa K. Tolba, executive director of the United Nations Environment Program, summed up the need for all of us to do what we can, **now**, while we still can, when he said, "There is not a single nation or individual on Earth whose well-being is not finally dependent on its biological resources, its seas and rivers, grasslands, forests, soil, and air. Unless all nations mount a massive and sustained effort into safeguarding their shared living resources, we would face a catastrophe only on a scale rivaled by nuclear war."[114]

Dr. Barry Commoner, who has been writing essays on environmental issues before it was as topical a subject as it is today, points out: "Now we are stealing from future generations not just their lumber or coal, but the basic necessities of life: air, water, soil. A new conservation movement is needed to preserve life itself."[115]

In the words of David Brower, past head of both the Sierra Club and Friends of the Earth, present head of Earth Island Institute, and a man considered by many preservationists to be the quintessential American conservationist, "Man's diminishing of the Earth is a crime, and the worst one of all is grand larceny against the future."[116]

The issue is no longer a question of whether or not we are putting ourselves and our children in peril, but rather, how we are going to stop doing it.

THERE'S NO LACK OF CONCERN

One thing is now quite certain: people are aware of and concerned with the plight of our planet's health. A Gallup poll indicated that 75 percent of Americans considered themselves to be environmentalists.[117] The poll stated that 72 percent of people "worry a great deal" about pollution of rivers, lakes, and reservoirs; 69 percent about contamination of soil and water by toxic wastes; and 63 percent about air pollution.

A Louis Harris poll of citizens and leaders of 15 countries showed that over 70 percent would be willing to pay higher taxes to protect the environment. In the U.S., it was over 80 percent.[118] **Higher taxes!**

Fortunately, we do not have to wait for the nations of the world to join together in a combined rescue effort, as I am sure they eventually will.

In the meantime, there is something that those people concerned with the environment can do **right now**:

Decrease your own animal products consumption. Our children—our planet—are depending on us all to do so.

VICTORY!

At the end of World War II, there was a symbol that became well known to one and all. People held up two fingers in the shape of a **V** to signify **V-Day**, the day of Victory.

We now have a new **V-Day** for the coming century—Vegetarian Day—and it is also a victory— a victory that has no losers, only winners.

Be a winner—support **V-Day!**

THE MORE THE MERRIER

As is true with any worthwhile project, there will be those who wish to do even more than reducing their consumption of animal products.

For those individuals, there are two activities that can greatly accelerate all of the positive results described above.

First, remember when the pyramid money scheme was all the rage? Participants paid $1,000 and recruited two others who also paid $1,000. Each new recruit brought in two more people, and in a matter of a few weeks, the first group walked away with a bundle of money. The pyramids were quickly outlawed, though, because while a few scored big, a lot of others lost. One thing this scheme did prove, though, was how a massive number of people could be reached in a very short period of time in order to accomplish something.

We can use that same concept to spread the **V-Day** message effectively and efficiently. During your once-a-week vegetarian day, you can bring the awareness of what you are doing and **why** to at least two other individuals who you believe would be open to participating in **V-Day**. They, too, can mobilize two others to join in the endeavor. Those two people can, in turn, do the same, and soon, the idea will spread throughout the country, resulting in a cleaner, healthier environment.

SPREAD THE WORD

If all you do is see to it that at least two other people have the opportunity to read this little book, you will be making a powerful contribution!

It is human nature to do good and to support worthy causes in order to bring about the **greater** good. Well, what cause is more worthy than helping to preserve life on Earth?

When you communicate the startling connection between our food choices and the health of our planet to friends and acquaintances who have not yet discovered this link, they will appreciate the fact that you've enabled them to get involved. This project is too important for anyone to be denied the opportunity to participate and make a difference.

"I THINK THAT I SHALL NEVER SEE A POEM LOVELY AS A TREE"

The second measure that we can take to get this project on a successful course is probably the most noble and gratifying of all:

PLANT TREES!

Wherever and whenever possible, plant a tree. Either personally, in your own backyard, or in support of those groups that are heading up tree-planting campaigns. **Presently, on a worldwide basis, we are cutting trees ten times faster than we are replanting them,**[119] so there is no time to waste on this one.

Every tree planted brings us one step closer to regaining a healthier carbon dioxide/oxygen balance. The sooner the carbon dioxide level in the atmosphere is lowered, the sooner we will find relief from the crisis of global warming caused by the greenhouse effect.

Every tree that is planted can neutralize the carbon dioxide produced by the burning of one ton of coal.[120]

EVERY TREE HELPS!

Prior to the 1984 Olympic games in Southern California, the Los Angeles-based, nonprofit group, TreePeople, joined with government agencies and private organizations to plant one million trees in time for the Olympics. A committed group of concerned citizens achieved this goal on a shoestring budget.

That effort became a model for groups around the world. Based on the Los Angeles effort, a campaign to plant **200 million trees** is just now coming to fruition in Australia. The TreePeople are presently inaugurating a campaign to plant 100 million trees in the United States.

Helping organizations such as TreePeople in any way not only helps the planet as a whole, but is a wonderful way to support the future of your own family and friends.

PLANTING THE SEED . . .

Right now, the American Forestry Association estimates that there are 100 million spaces where additional trees can be planted around American homes and communities. The planting of urban trees is one of the most cost-effective techniques to significantly affect the total imbalance in the transfer of carbon dioxide from earth to air.[121] It is something that can be done immediately, by ordinary citizens and local organizations.

For every ton of timber created as a result of a tree's growth, one-and-a-half tons of carbon dioxide are absorbed, and one ton of oxygen is released.[122]

One hundred million trees planted will reduce carbon dioxide emissions by **18 million tons a year**[123] **while releasing 12 million tons of oxygen.**[124]

Studies by scientists at the Lawrence Livermore Laboratories show that simply planting three trees around a house—two on the south side and one on the west side—could save as much as 44 percent of the energy required to cool an average household.[125] The total effect, in terms of reduced power demands and energy consumption, can translate into a significant impact on national carbon dioxide reduction goals. People can reduce energy consumption and plant trees simultaneously.

The Lawrence Livermore Laboratories also report that a properly placed city tree absorbs 30 times as much carbon dioxide as a forest tree, thereby helping to fight global warming while reducing energy demands.[126]

Scientists estimate that improving the woodlands could remove as much as one-third of the total carbon dioxide now being released into the air by the burning of fossil fuels.[127]

IF NOT NOW—WHEN?

If we start planting **right now**, in the words of R. Neil Sampson, executive vice president of the American Forestry Association, and a man whose dedication to the forests is unwavering, "we'll enter the 21st century with millions of trees that have been growing for a decade, gaining in size, beauty, and value. We'll have millions of people who recognized a serious threat and took the appropriate action."[128]

It is my hope that every person who reads this book will become a member of the American Forestry Association (see page 208). The A.F.A. has championed the protection and building of forests for over 100 years. Their Global ReLeaf program is proving to be one of the most ambitious and successful tree-planting campaigns in the country. Its bimonthly magazine, *American Forests*, is invaluable.

In addition to the American Forestry Association, the TreePeople, (see page 216) are ready, willing, and able to give advice on all aspects of tree planting, including types of trees, age of trees, the best time to plant, location of trees, etc.

It all comes down to priorities. We are talking about the three basic requirements of life: air, water, and food, all provided for by our environment. Yet we have spent more on weapons in the last **six hours** than we have spent on the environment in the last **ten years!**[129] Military spending, worldwide, is 2.5 billion dollars **a day.**[130] The world's stockpile of nuclear weapons is equivalent to 3.2 tons of dynamite for every man, woman, and child on Earth.[131]

Considering some of the recent encouraging developments in the world (Gorbachev's *Perestroika*, destruction of the Berlin Wall, etc.), a very convincing argument could be made for redefining security and reordering priorities to divert some of that two-and-a-half billion dollars a day toward a more imminent problem: the planet's ill health.

IF WE ALL PULL TOGETHER AS A TEAM

What we are attempting to accomplish here is more than a labor of love, it is a labor of **life**. This is not an issue that is Democrat or Republican, male or female, black or white, Christian or Jew, American, European, or Asian. It is an issue for anyone who breathes!

The threat to our very existence **can** be successfully thwarted, but only if we act. We are in danger only if we do nothing. Surely it is no crime to attempt to do something and not succeed. The crime is in not even trying.

Ultimately, the nurturing and healing that our planet is now so direly in need of is going to come not from the commitment of one nation to another, but from the commitment of human beings to Earth.

As Pope John Paul II so eloquently stated, protecting the environment and limiting damage already inflicted, is the responsibility of "the entire human community."[132]

It is not my intention to give the impression that we merely have to reduce animal product production and consumption to see the problems threatening our environment magically disappear. We all know that there are too many factors, too many variables, for that to be the case. The dizzying array and quantity of toxic chemicals produced over the last 50 years have practically saturated our environment.

Automobiles and power plants spew billions of tons of fumes into the air and create the acid rain we now must endure. Gargantuan accumulations of garbage are dumped into landfills and waterways. The spectre of nuclear proliferation, with its potential for accidents of devastating proportions, looms over us. The fact is, it would be a formidable challenge to compile a list of all the problems we are facing, with all their potential solutions.

However, when we speak of the production of America's meat-based diet, we are talking about something that **does** massively impact our environment. Here is an opportunity that allows the individual to take meaningful action, as opposed to having to deal with the feeling of helplessness that arises from not knowing whether or not those in control will do the right thing.

LIGHT AT THE END OF THE TUNNEL

Now, after devoting so much time to the alarming issues that demand our attention, we would be doing ourselves a disservice if we did not explore all the **good** that is being done for our environment as well.

Many of us feel the need to **do something** wherever something can be done, and this sensitivity to the call for action is making a difference:

How We're All Helping

1. Recycling is becoming more and more common. Paper, bottles, plastics, and cans are all being recycled.* Japan presently recycles over 50 percent of its trash. Western Europe and the United States recycle 30 percent and 10

---

*Paper recycling can have wonderfully positive repercussions. The U.S. is the world's largest consumer of paper, using 600 pounds per capita a year.[133] Not only does recycled paper require 64 percent less energy to produce, but it also results in 74 percent less air pollution and 35 percent less water pollution.[134] And, of course, recycling paper saves our forests. Every ton of recycled paper produced saves approximately 17 trees.[135]

percent respectively.[136] At least 30 states in the U.S. are in the process of implementing some kind of trash separation program for recycling.[137]

2. Carpooling has cut back on the number of cars on the road, reducing fuel use.

3. Homeowners are insulating walls and ceilings and wrapping hot water heaters in blanket insulation. Both save fuel, thereby sharply reducing the amount of carbon dioxide released into the atmosphere.

4. There is a new awareness about the damage caused by styrofoam. One of the many ways that people can avoid the use of styrofoam is to bring reusable cups to work, instead of taking another styrofoam cup each time they want something to drink.

5. Many efforts are being made to save water. Fixing leaky faucets, placing a brick in toilet tanks or obtaining low-flush toilets, sweeping sidewalks and driveways instead of washing them down, watering lawns at night rather than when the sun is shining in order to cut down on evaporation are all commonly practiced water conservation measures.

6. Turning off lights not in use is done with regularity.

7. Compact fluorescent light bulbs are being used to replace incandescent bulbs because they use far less energy.

8. Tremendous progress has been made in the household cleaning industry. Standard household cleaning aids (generally made from petroleum products, artificial colors and fragrances) and irritating and environmentally harmful bleaches are rapidly being replaced by ecologically safe alternatives.

We are now more conscious of the fact that the toxic products we have been using break down very slowly and oftentimes incompletely, thus contributing to the pollution of our rivers, lakes, bays, and oceans. Many of us are switching to 100 percent biodegradable products that break down into harmless natural substances within 3 to 5 days.*

---

*A variety of these products can be acquired through the "Seventh Generation Catalog," 10 Farrell St., S. Burlington, Vermont 05403, 800/456-1177.

9. There is ongoing research to perfect the use of methanol, ethanol, and hydrogen for automobiles. In fact, there are some cars now using them as fuel, although these are still very few in number. We can see, however, that the technology exists, and is improving.

10. At landfills where it exists, methane gas is being trapped and used. This gas generates one-half the carbon dioxide that coal generates, while producing the same amount of energy.[138]

11. The technology for solar energy, which generates **no** waste and is literally an inexhaustible source of energy, is becoming more sophisticated and more affordable every day. The cost of solar photovoltaic cells has dropped 75 percent since 1980.[139]

12. Tree planting has caught on. There are projects all over the world to reforest the land. In many cities in the United States, both government and private corporations are sponsoring tree-planting campaigns. In his State of the Union Address in January of 1990, President George Bush pledged to allocate sufficient funds to plant one billion trees a

year across the U.S. In Australia, Prime Minister Bob Hawke has called for a new national program to plant one billion trees by the year 2000.

13. Many people are heeding the suggestions of leading experts to cut back on their beef intake. In 1970, Americans ate an average of 114 pounds of beef per person. In 1988, we saw a significant drop, to 70 pounds per person.[140]

    A recent Gallup Poll said that up to 45 percent of Americans are eliminating red meat from their diets, and 36 percent are cutting out dairy foods.[140A]

14. Eighty-one nations, including the United States and Russia, have adopted a declaration calling for a complete phase-out of chlorofluorocarbons (CFCs).[141]

15. Although toxic wastes have, up until recently, been recklessly dumped just about **anywhere** —in lakes, streams, back lots, swamps—that practice is increasingly being policed and curtailed. Many countries have cleaned up acres of waste, and strategies to control the volume of waste are being formulated.

16. There are national and international efforts to clean up the waterways. Only a few years ago, Lake Michigan and Lake Erie could not support the life of a single fish. Today both bodies of water are supporting an ever-growing fish population.

17. Composting of trash into soil, which used to receive scant, if any, attention, has been discovered. In 1989 the number of trash-composting projects in the United States increased by almost 80 percent.[142]

18. Many hundreds of farmers all over the United States are either switching to organic farming methods or investigating this practice. Spurring on this enormously positive trend is the ever-growing number of individuals who are actively seeking organically grown food to avoid the harmful chemicals so routinely dumped on the land and the crops it produces, and a National Academy of Sciences report, which found that organic farming is usually as productive as farming with pesticides and synthetic fertilizers.[143]

19. Corporate America has begun to do its part now that it has learned that it is possible to do

well by doing good. According to Fortune Magazine, major companies throughout the United States are making major changes that will bring their products to market in a far more environmentally friendly way than ever before.[144]

20. The World Bank, which lends money for Third World development projects, is increasingly withholding funds from ecologically unsound programs. The result is a heightened public awareness of environmental issues and a new entrepreneurial interest in environmentally sound projects. The World Bank recently declared its intention to raise its funding for studies to preserve tropical rainforests from $138 million to $350 million by 1990.[145]

21. In what is called a "Debt-for-Nature-Swap," a $5.6 million Costa Rican debt to American Express bank was purchased for $748,000 by the Nature Conservancy and several donors, in exchange for the protection of 355,000 acres of Costa Rican habitat. A similar arrangement was made in Ecuador for a $9 million debt. In Bolivia a $650,000 debt was cancelled in exchange for a promise to conserve nearly three million acres of forest and grassland. Other

such debt-for-swap transactions are presently under way.

22. Eight nations of South America's Amazon basin have joined together to protect their rainforests. The presidents of Brazil, Colombia, Ecuador, Guyana, Peru, Suriname, and Venezuela, and the Foreign Minister of Bolivia, have met and issued a "Declaration of Amazonia" in response to "the world outcry over the onslaught on the forests."[146]

23. The political party, Greens (see page 212), which started in Europe and is totally committed to the ecology of planet Earth, has become a worldwide movement. Greens have been elected to national parliaments in Switzerland, Belgium, West Germany, Finland, Austria, Italy, Luxembourg, Sweden, Portugal, and Iceland.[147] More than 3,000 Greens sit in federal, state, and local lawmaking bodies in West Germany alone.[148] The movement is becoming increasingly popular in the United States.

24. There is an increasingly popular movement throughout the world called "green consumerism." It refers to making informed choices

188

before buying a particular product. The Council on Economic Priorities (CEP) publishes a booklet* pointing out which companies harm the environment in the process of bringing their products to market and which ones do not. For example, Safeway and Quaker Oats receive high marks, while American Cyanimid and Squibb do not. This type of information gives us all a chance to use the "power of the purse" to convince companies to conduct business in a more socially responsible fashion.

*Shopping For A Better World—A Quick and Easy Guide to Socially Responsible Supermarket Shopping. CEP, 30 Irving Place, New York City, N.Y. 10003 (800) 822-6435.

AND FURTHERMORE . . .

William Reilly, president of the Wildlife Fund, has been appointed head of the Environmental Protection Agency (EPA). Mr. Reilly has wasted no time. In addition to the recommendation to end CFC use, proposed EPA measures include:

- A halt to "net global deforestation" by planting as many new trees as those felled.
- A set of fees (taxes) on coal, oil, and natural gas aimed at providing incentives to shift away from fossil fuel use.
- Accelerated research on solar power (U.S. funds for solar research over the last eight years have been considerably reduced).
- A sharp increase in the use of biomass fuels (i.e., trees) vs. fossil fuels.
- A program to increase the efficiency of home heating, aimed at reducing the amount of fuel used per home to one-half the 1980 level.[149]

Mr. Reilly's proposals are considerably more significant than the EPA's suggestions of just two years ago: offering sunscreens, sunglasses, and hats as a solution to ozone depletion!

As you can see, many encouraging trends are being established. Since we are all in this effort together, we are beginning to see that when all of us are willing to do our part, a significant amount of progress can be made. It is comforting to know that when it really counts, so many concerned citizens can be mobilized to action.

YES! I WANT TO DO MY PART

Whether you are a person consumed by the subject of the environment—spending practically all of your waking hours on projects that will repair it—or someone who is only remotely aware of the need to do something, one thing is absolutely certain: By decreasing your consumption of animal products, you are part of the solution, not part of the problem. You are making a difference. A positive one. And there is no better time to make that difference than right now.

In the words of historian Thomas Carlyle: "Our grand business is not to see what lies dimly at a distance, but to do what lies clearly at hand."

Once again, thank you for taking the time. Thank you for caring.

Keep a fire for the human race,
Let your prayers go drifting into space,
You'll never know what will be coming down.

Perhaps a better world is drawing near,
Or just as easy we could all disappear,
Along with whatever meaning you might
   have found.

Don't let the uncertainty turn you around,
The world keeps turning around and around,
Don't it make a joyous sound!

—Jackson Browne
(from ''For a Dancer'')

NOTES

1. The Surgeon General's "Report on Nutrition and Health," U.S. Dept. of Health and Human Services, 1988.

2. American Heart Association, as noted in *Los Angeles Times*, January 17, 1989.

3. Op. cit. note 1.

4. "The Dismal Truth About Teen-Age Health," *Reader's Digest*, March, 1986.

4A. Marlene Cimons, "U.S. Urges Cholesterol Cut Even If Disease Risk Is Low," *L.A. Times*, February 28, 1990.

5. *L.A. Times*, September 24, 1989.

6. Thomas H. Maugh II, "Ocean Data Shows Global Warming May Have Begun," *L.A. Times*, April 20, 1989.

7. "First Evidence of Solar Icecap Melting," *The Environment Digest*, No. 29, October, 1989.

8. Michael Parrish, "Rising Sea Seeping Into Coast Plans," *L.A. Times*, August 15, 1989.

9. Ibid.

10. *L.A. Times*, May 25, 1989.

11. "Feeling the Heat," *Time*, January 2, 1989.

12. "Growing Concern Over Global Warming," *The Animal's Voice*, Vol. 2, No. 2, April, 1989.

13. Michael Rogers, "Five Weathermen of the Apocalypse," *L.A. Times Magazine*, May 21, 1989.

14. "The Drought of '89: World Food Supplies Are Dwindling Fast," *Solstice*, Issue #35, March/April, 1989.

NOTES, cont'd.

15. "Breadbaskets And Dustbowls," *Solstice*, Vol. 36, May/June, 1989.

16. Ibid.

17. Elizabeth Darby-Junkin, "Environment As National Security," *Buzzworm*, Summer, 1989.

18. Op. cit. note 14.

19. Michael Satchell, "The Whole Earth Agenda," *U.S. News & World Report*, December 25, 1989–January 1, 1990.

20. Larry B. Stammer, "Saving the Earth: Who Sacrifices?" *Los Angeles Times*, March 13, 1989.

21. Richard Monestersky, "Global Change: The Scientific Challenge," *Science News*, Vol. 135, No. 15, April 15, 1989.

22. Art Pine, "Summit Stresses Ecological Threat," *L.A. Times*, July 17, 1989.

23. Tom Regan, "But For The Sake Of Some Little Mouthful Of Flesh," *The Animal's Agenda*, Vol. 2, No. 1, February, 1989.

24. "The Global Bonfire," *New York Times*, July 1, 1989.

    Neil R. Sampson, "ReLeaf For Global Warming," *American Forests*, November/December, 1988.

25. David Pimental, "Hot Wiring America's Farms," *Fueling The Future*, aired on PBS January 17, 1989.

26. Hodding Carter, Op. cit. note 25.

27. Drew DeSilver, "The Cattle-Drought Connection," *Vegetarian Times*, July, 1989.

28. U.S.D.A. chart, as illustrated in "Our Common Future: Healing the Planet," symposium organized by UCLA School of Medicine, May 13, 1989.

29. Mary Bralove, "The Food Crisis: The Shortages May Pit the 'Have Nots' Against the 'Haves'," *Wall Street Journal*, October 3, 1974.

    Op. cit. note 34, Table 6 I 1.

    U.S.D.A., *Agricultural Statistics*, 1984.

NOTES, cont'd.

30. H.J. Maidenburg, "The Livestock Explosion," *New York Times*, July 1, 1973.

    Op. cit. note 33, Table 203 and 1983 Table 205.

    Op. cit. note 34.

    U.S.D.A., *Agricultural Statistics*, 1984.

31. Mary Bralove, Op. cit. note 29.

32. U.S.D.A., *Agricultural Statistics*, 1984.

    U.S.D.A., "Composition of Foods," Table 6, 1963.

    Op. cit. note 34.

33. *Statistical Abstract of the United States*, Exhibits #1211 and 1221, 1982–1983.

34. *Soil and Water Resources Conservation Act*, Review Draft Part I, Appraisal 1980, United States Department of Agriculture.

    Personal conversation with Robin Hur.

34A. National Agriculture Land Study, National Resources Inventory, 1982.

    Agricultural Statistics, United States Department of Agriculture, 1981 and 1988.

    Op. cit. note 34.

34B. Ibid.

    Statistical Abstract of the United States, U.S. Department of Agriculture, Chart #1148, 1982–1983.

35. *Commercial Fertilizer Consumption in the United States*, U.S.D.A. Statistical Reporting Service, 1985.

36. John Cogan, Energy Information Center, Department of Energy, Washington, D.C., via personal communication, February 26, 1990.

    Frank Maxey, Energy Specialist, Office of Chemicals and Applied Products, U.S. Department of Commerce, Washington, D.C., via personal communication, February 26, 1990.

NOTES, cont'd.

37. S. Harris, "Organichlorine Contamination of Breast Milk," *Environmental Defense Fund*, Washington, D.C., November 7, 1979.

    J. Balbien; S. Harris; and T. Page, "Diet as a Factor Affecting Organichlorine Contamination of Breast Milk," *Environmental Defense Fund*, Washington, D.C.

38. Frances Moore Lappé, *Diet for a Small Planet*, Tenth Anniversary Edition, (New York: Ballantine Books, 1982).

    Alan Durning, Worldwatch Institute researcher.

39. Ibid.

40. "The Browning of America," *Newsweek*, February 22, 1981.

41. Georg Borgstrom, Presentation to the Annual Meeting of the American Association for the Advancement of Science.

    Paul and Anne Ehrlich, *Population, Resources, Environment*, (W. H. Freeman, 1972).

42. Marc Reisner, "The Emerald Desert," *Greenpeace*, Vol. 14, No. 4, July/August, 1989.

43. Op. cit. note 51, John Robbins.

44. William Lagrone, "The Great Plains," in *Another Revolution in U.S. Farming?* Schertz, et al., U.S.D.A., E.S.C.S., Agricultural Economic Report No. 41, December, 1979.

    "Report: Nebraska's Water Wealth Is Deceptive," *Omaha World Hearald*, May 28, 1981.

    John Seymour and Herbert Girardet, *Blueprint for a Green Planet*, Prentice-Hall, New York, 1987.

45. *Soil and Water Resources Conservation Act*, 1980 Appraisal Review Draft, Part I, U.S. Dept. of Agriculture.

    Georg Borgstrom, cited in *Diet For A Small Planet*, 1975 Edition.

    Raymond Loehr, *Pollution Implications of Animal Wastes*, Water Pollution Control Research Series, Washington, D.C., Office of Research Monitoring, U.S.E.P.A., 1968.

46. Jim Mason and Pete Singer, *Animal Factories*, (New York: Crown Publishers, 1980).

NOTES, cont'd.

David Pimental, "Energy and Land Constraints in Food Protein Production," *Science*, November 21, 1975.

H.A. Jasiorowski, "Intensive Systems of Animal Production," *Proceedings of the Third World Conference on Animal Production*, ed. R.F. Reid, Sydney University Press, 1975.

Jackie Robbins, *Environmental Impact Resulting From Unconfined Animal Production*, Environmental Protection Technology Series, Cincinnati, U.S.E.P.A., Office of Research and Development, Environmental Research Information Center, February, 1978.

47. Bruce Myles, "U.S. Antipollution Laws May Boost Cattle Feeders' Costs and Meat Prices," *Christian Science Monitor*, March 11, 1974.

48. Op. cit. note 117.

    Op. cit. note 118.

49. Op. cit. note 34.

    Agricultural Statistics, U.S.D.A., 1984.

50. "The World Food Problem," A Report By *The President's Science Advisory Committee*, Vol. II, May, 1967.

    Fact Sheet, *Food Animals Concern Trust*, Issue 26, November, 1982, Chicago.

51. John Robbins, *Diet For A New America* (Walpole, N.H.: Stillpoint Publishing, 1987).

    Aaron Altschul, *Proteins: Their Chemistry and Politics* (Basic Books, 1965).

    Folke Dovring, "Soybeans," *Scientific American*, February, 1974.

52. S. Nelson, "Non-Dietary Factors in Nutrition," *The Life Science Health System*, College of Life Science, Austin, Texas, 1978.

53. N. Mead, J.D. Mann, and D. Yarrow, "Whither the Trees?" *Solstice*, Issue #34, December/January, 1989.

    Lester Brown, foreword to Perlin, John, *A Forest Journey* (New York: W.W. Norton, 1989).

NOTES, cont'd.

Sandra Postel, "Global View of a Tropical Disaster," *American Forests*, November/December, 1988.

54. Robin Hur and Dr. David Fields, "Are High-Fat Diets Killing Our Forests?" *Vegetarian Times*, February, 1984.

55. Ibid.

56. Neil R. Sampson, "ReLeaf for Global Warming," *American Forests*, November/December, 1988.

57. Op. cit. note 54.

58. "Life In the Balance," aired on PBS, March 29, 1989.

59. Neil R. Sampson, "Cool the Greenhouse, Plant 100 Million Trees," *Los Angeles Times*, October 16, 1988.

60. Susan Meeker-Lowry, "Saving the Rainforests: An Economist's Plan," *Organica*, Vol. 8, No. 27, Spring, 1989.

61. Aubrey Hampton, "Saving the Rainforests is Saving Ourselves," *Organica*, Vol. 8, No. 27, Spring, 1989.

62. "Hamburgers are Killing Trees," *Newsweek*, September 14, 1987.

63. Ibid.

64. John Robbins, Op. cit. note 51.

Acres, U.S.A., Kansas City, Mo. Vol. 16, No. 6, June, 1985.

65. Op. cit. note 74.

66. James Parsons, "Forest to Pasture: Development or Destruction?" *Revista De Biologia Tropical*, Volume 24, Supp. No. 1, 1976.

67. Philip M. Fearnside, "Deforestation In Brazilian Amazonia," *The Earth In Transition: Patterns and Processes of Biotic Impoverishment*, Cambridge University Press, 1990.

68. John David Mann and David Yarrow, "Diets and Deeds of Dinosaurs," *Solstice*, Issue #34, December/January, 1989.

69. Op. cit. note 24.

70. Op. cit. note 60.

NOTES, cont'd.

71. Randall Hayes, "Gone With The Trees," *The Animal's Voice*, Vol. 2, No. 1, February, 1989.

    David Suzuki, "The Biosphere Dwarfs Other Issues," *Earth Island Journal*, Fall, 1989.

72. Dick Russell, "The Critical Decade," *E: The Environmental Magazine*, Vol. 1, No. 1, January/February, 1990.

73. "Life in the Balance," aired on PBS April 11, 1989.

74. "Rediscovering Planet Earth," *U.S. News and World Report*, October 31, 1988. (Actual research was conducted by Christopher Uhl, assistant professor of biology, Penn State University.)

75. Ibid.

75A. Judy Krizmanic, "Why Cutting Out Meat Can Cool the Earth," *Vegetarian Times*, No. 152, April, 1990.

76. "Crimes Against Nature," *Earth Island Journal*, Spring, 1989.

77. Karl Schoenberger, "A Lust for Trees, A Love of Wood," *L.A. Times*, December 20, 1989.

78. "Malaysia's Forests Are Going Fast," *Earth Island Journal*, Spring, 1989.

79. "Japan Plan To Pave The Andes, *Earth Island Journal*, Spring, 1989.

80. "Rainforests," *The Environmental Digest*, No. 25, June, 1989.

81. Edward A. Hansen, *Energy Plantations in North Central United States: Status of Research and Development Plantations*, United States Dept. of Agriculture, Forest Service, Rhinelander, Wisconsin, 1988.

82. "Have Your Rainforest and Eat It Too," *Science News*, Vol. 136, No. 3, July 15, 1989.

83. Eugene Linden, "Playing with Fire," *Time*, September 18, 1989.

84. Op. cit. note 72.

85. Vernon G. Carter and Tom Dale, *Topsoil and Civilization*, (University of Oklahoma Press, 1974).

NOTES, cont'd.

H. W. Lawton and P. T. Wilke, "Ancient Agriculture Systems In Dry Regions," in A. E. Hall, G. H. Cannell, and H. W. Lawton, *Agriculture In Semi Arid Environments*, Springer-Verlag, N.Y., 1979.

86. William Brune, State Conservationist, Soil Conservation Service, Des Moines, Iowa; testimony before Senate Committee on Agriculture and Forestry, July 6, 1976.

    Seth King, "Iowa Rain and Wind Deplete Farm Lands," *New York Times*, December 5, 1976.

    Curtis Harnack, "In Plymouth County, Iowa, the Rich Topsoil's Going Fast, Alas," *New York Times*, July 11, 1980.

87. Robin Hur, "Six Inches From Starvation: How and Why America's Topsoil is Disappearing," *Vegetarian Times*, March, 1985.

    David Pimental, et al., "Land Degradation: Effects On Food and Energy," *Science*, Volume 194, October, 1976.

    National Association of Conservation Districts, Washington, D.C., *Soil Degradation: Effects On Agricultural Productivity*, Interim Report No. 4, National Agricultural Lands Study, 1980.

    Seth King, "Farms Go Down The River," *New York Times*, December 10, 1978.

88. Robin Hur, Op. cit. note 87.

89. Op. cit. note 44, John Seymour.

90. David Pimental, et. al, *Advances In Food Research*, Vol. 32, Academic Press, 1988.

91. "Soil and Water Resources Conservation Act—Summary of Appraisal," U.S.D.A. Review Draft, 1980.

    David Pimental, Op. cit. note 87.

    National Association of Conservation Districts, Op. cit. note 87.

    U.S.D.A., Economics and Statistics Service, *Natural Resource Capital in U.S. Agriculture: Irrigation, Drainage, and Conservation Investments Since 1900*, E.S.C.S. Staff Paper, March, 1979.

NOTES, cont'd.

92. Op. cit. note 54.

Op. cit. note 32.

Conversation between Robin Hur and:
K. Miller and J. Dose, Bureau of Land Management, U.S. Dept. of Interior, Washington, D.C.;
W. Evans, D. Funking and J. Perry, National Forest Service, Washington, D.C.; and
R. Wolf, Library of Congress, Washington, D.C.

93. Dyan Zaslowsky, "A Public Beef: Are Grazing Cattle Turning The American West Into A New Desert?" *Harrowsmith*, January/February, 1989.

94. Ibid.

95. Ibid.

96. Op. cit. note 27.

97. Ibid.

98. Op. cit. note 93.

99. Ibid.

100. Ibid.

101. Mark A. Stein and Louis Sahagun, "BLM Woes Spill Onto Public Lands" and "Environment Activists Hit Bush Choice for U.S. Post," *L.A. Times*, May 21, 1989.

"Ranchers Turn A Profit by Subletting U.S. Land," *L.A. Times*, May 23, 1989.

102. Ibid.

103. "Will We Mend Our Earth?" *National Geographic*, Vol. 174, No. 6, December, 1988.

104. *Statistical Abstract of the United States*, 103rd Edition, 1982-1983, United States Dept. of Commerce, Bureau of Census, Table #344.

105. Op. cit. note 45.

106. Robin Hur and David Fields, "How Meat Robs America of Its Energy," *Vegetarian Times*, April, 1985.

NOTES, cont'd.

J. T. Reid, "Comparative Efficiency of Animals in the Conversion of Feedstuffs to Human Foods," *Confinement*, April, 1976.

W. L. Roller, et al., "Energy Costs of Intensive Livestock Production," American Society of Agricultural Engineers, June, 1975, St. Joseph, Michigan, Paper No. 75-4042, Table 7.

The research for note 106 was done by Robin Hur. Information was garnered from a vast number of government organizations and private trade organizations. Some notable ones were The National Agricultural Land Study, U.S. Department of Agriculture, Department of Energy, Department of Transportation, Bureau of Economic Analysis, Bureau of the Census, Federal Highway Administration, and the Oak Ridge National Laboratories.

107. Robin Hur, Op. cit. note 54, and as per personal conversation.

108. Lester Brown, (of) The Overseas Development Council, as cited in *Diet For A New America*, 1987.

109. "World Hunger," Report by the Food and Agricultural Organization of the United Nations (FAO) in Rome, Italy, Fall, 1989.

110. Op. cit. note 86.

111. Op. cit. note 34.

112. Op. cit. note 23.

113. "What On Earth Are We Doing," *Time*, January 2, 1989.

114. "A Truce With Earth," *Los Angeles Times*, March 13, 1989.

115. Richard Grossman, "Of Time and Tide," *Earth Island Journal*, Spring, 1989.

116. Brandon Mitchener, "Out On A Limb For Mother Earth," *E: The Environmental Magazine*, Vol. 1, No.1, January/February 1990.

117. *L.A. Times*, May 17, 1989.

118. "Alarums! Cries New World Poll," *Environmental Action*, July/August, 1989.

119. Russell Peterson, "At Last, Earth's Future Is A Truly Global Concern," *L.A. Times*, May 14, 1989.

NOTES, cont'd.

120. "Keep Greenhouse At Bay," *Greenpeace*, Vol. 14, No. 4, July/August, 1989.

121. Op. cit. note 59.

122. Donald J. Nichol, *Trees: Guardians of the Earth*, (Washington: Morningtown Press, 1988).

123. Op. cit. note 17.

124. Op. cit. note 122.

125. "Tree Power," *Earth Island Journal*, Winter, 1988–89.

126. Ibid.

127. Op. cit. note 59.

128. Ibid.

129. *Discovery Program*, "The State of the Planet," aired November 25, 1985.

130. Op. cit. note 17.

131. "World Military and Social Expenditures," U.S. Department of Defense, 1982.

132. William D. Montalbano, "Pope Warns of Global Ecological Crisis," *L.A. Times*, December 6, 1989.

133. Op. cit. note 60.

134. Thomas H. Rawls, "Ordinary People," *Harrowsmith*, No. 25, January/February, 1990.

135. "The Challenge Now," *ORION: Nature Quarterly*, Winter, 1990.

136. "A Stinking Mess," *Time*, January 2, 1989.

137. Op. cit. note 72.

138. "Feeling the Heat," Time, January 2, 1989.

139. "The Sun Shines On A Brave Renewable World," *Earth Island Journal*, Summer, 1989.

140. "The Sweet Smell of Success," *Harrowsmith*, January/February, 1989.

"Red Meat Is No Longer Rare On Restaurant Menus," *USA Today*, August 8, 1989.

NOTES, cont'd.

140A. "Simple Guidelines to Develop a More Healthful Diet," *L.A. Times*, March 15, 1990.

141. "Call For Stronger Ozone Protection," *Science News*, Vol. 135, No. 23, June 10, 1989.

142. Michael Parrish, "Trash Idea Rises From the Heap," *L.A. Times*, February 8, 1990.

143. *L.A. Times*, September 9, 1989.

144. David Kirkpatrick, "Environmentalism: The New Crusade," *Fortune*, February 12, 1990.

145. Timothy C. Weiskel, "The Ecological Lessons of the Past: An Anthropology of Environmental Decline," *The Ecologist*, Vol. 19, No. 3, May/June, 1989.

146. *L.A. Times*, May 7, 1989.

147. William D. Montalbano, "Green Wave Surging Over West Europe," *L.A. Times*, May 11, 1989.

148. Ibid.

149. "The Greenhousing Of Politics," *Solstice*, Vol. 36, May/June, 1989.

RECOMMENDED RESOURCES

I designed this book to be highly focused and easy to read. It's difficult to include everything I'd like to share with you—thus, the inclusion here of a selected list of organizations, publications, and books. I have personally found them all to be helpful, informative, and truly dedicated to our personal and planetary health. Of course, it is impossible to list every relevant resource, for there are so many people and groups involved in the environmental movement, and more join the ranks every day. So I may have missed something inadvertently.

However, the list of organizations and published material that follows is a good start, and I trust you'll make your own special additions to it. I personally welcome your comments and suggestions for expanding and/or revising this list.

—Harvey Diamond

ORGANIZATIONS

Unless otherwise indicated, membership information refers to a one-year basic membership package. FAX numbers listed have the same area codes as main telephone numbers, except where the main number is a toll-free (800) number. Membership figures include both members and supporters.

THE AMERICAN FORESTRY ASSOCIATION, P.O. Box 2000, Washington, D.C. 20013, (800) 368-5748, President: Richard M. Hollier, Jr. Founded in 1875 by a group of horticulturists, the AFA has 80,000 members. Its concerns include all issues related to trees, forests, and forestry. Its focus is to improve, maintain, expand, and enhance the health and value of trees. It is America's oldest citizen-membership conservation group, and provides a wealth of information upon request. Membership: $24, includes the beautifully produced *American Forests* magazine.

BETTER WORLD SOCIETY, P.O. Box 96051, Washington, D.C. 20077, (800) 543-8000; FAX: (212) 692-6902, Executive Director: Thomas S. Belford. Founded in 1985 by Ted Turner (the force behind Turner Broadcasting System), this 28,000-member group's mission is to harness the power of television to make a better world. It raises funds by donation and membership to produce programs with environmental and human rights content. To that end, it has funded many such programs to date. Its international board of directors includes current and former heads of state and highly regarded environmentalists. Ted Turner's contribution in this area truly qualifies him as one of America's heroes. Membership: $20, includes newsletter.

THE CLIMATE INSTITUTE, 316 Pennsylvania Avenue, SE, Suite 403, Washington, D.C. 20003, (202) 547-0104; FAX: (202) 547-0111, President: John C. Topping, Jr. Founded in 1986, this organization acts as a link between scientists, governments, private decision-makers, and the public, regarding greenhouse warming and stratospheric ozone depletion. It holds conferences on those and related topics, offers workshops, and produces publications. Membership: $35, includes *Climate Alert* newsletter.

CONSERVATION INTERNATIONAL, 1015 Eighteenth Street, NW, Suite 1000, Washington, D.C. 20036, (202) 429-5660; FAX: (202) 887-5188, President: Dr. Russell A. Mittermeier. Founded in 1987 by 48 staff members of the Nature Conservancy, with 50,000 members, CI's mission is to develop the capacity to sustain biological diversity and the ecosystems and processes that support life on earth. It instituted the first debt-for-nature exchange in Bolivia, and it works with indigenous people, private and government organizations, especially in tropical areas of the Western Hemisphere. CI publishes *Tropicus, The Debt for Nature Exchange* and *Orion* magazine (in association with The Myrin Institute). Membership: $25, includes *Tropicus* quarterly newsletter.

THE COUSTEAU SOCIETY, 930 West Twenty-First Street, Norfolk, VA 23517, (804) 627-1144; FAX: (804) 627-7547, President: Jacques-Yves Cousteau. Founded in 1973, this extraordinary research and exploration organization now has 320,000 members. It serves to further the work of Jacques Cousteau and to educate the public about natural ecosystems. It publishes the *Calypso Log* and the *Dolphin Log* (for children), and produces at least four hours of new television programming each year. It also offers an annual program, "Project Ocean Search," to allow individuals to personally investigate one ecosystem with Cousteau's staff. Membership: $20, includes *Calypso Log*.

EARTH FIRST!, P.O. Box 5871, Tucson, AZ 85703, (602) 622-1371, Founders: Dave Foreman, Mike Roselle, et al. Created in 1981 by Dave Foreman and several other militant environmentalists, Earth

Earth First! (Continued)

First! is generally recognized to be an organization of aggressively passionate "ecowarriors." They say that their special brand of individual action is necessary to bring quick focus and needed change to various ecological problem areas. However, now that we are beginning to see tangible signs of environmental progress, perhaps some of what has frustrated Earth First! in the past will be allayed, and they can begin to revise their more combative (sometimes dangerous) tactics in favor of more temperate activities. Although there is no official membership structure, one can link up with the organization by subscribing to *Earth First! Journal* ($20)—an outspoken and very informative publication—published eight times a year and filled with ideas to help you participate in the solution of problems. They also have over 100 groups throughout the world that you can join.

EARTH ISLAND INSTITUTE, 300 Broadway, Suite 28, San Francisco, CA 94133, (415) 788-3666; FAX: (415) 788-7324, President: Ellen Manchester. Founded in 1982 by David R. Brower (first executive director of the Sierra Club and founder of Friends of the Earth), Earth Island develops and provides organizational support for innovative environmental projects. Current groups number 22 and include the Green Committees of Correspondence and marine mammal and rainforest projects. The Institute has over 25,000 members and publishes *Earth Island Journal*, a comprehensive quarterly newsmagazine that is well worth reading. Membership: $25, includes *Earth Island Journal.*

EARTHSAVE, 706 Frederick Street, Santa Cruz, CA 95062, (408) 423-4069; FAX: (408) 458-0255, Executive Director: Patricia Carney. Founded in 1988 by author and environmentalist John Robbins, this intensely committed group's mission is to educate the public about the dangers to the environment of meat-based agriculture and dietstyle, and to raise global environmental awareness. All profits from copies purchased through EarthSave of Robbins' book, *Diet for a New America*, go to the organization. Membership: $35, includes newsletter and updates.

ENVIRONMENTAL ACTION FOUNDATION, 1525 New Hampshire Avenue, NW, Washington, D.C. 20036, (202) 745-4870; FAX: (202) 745-4880, Executive Director: Ruth Caplan. Founded in 1970, this organization is composed of two arms. The foundation, funded by private donations and grants, provides information on environmental issues. Environmental Action, Inc., is a membership organization (20,000 members) that lobbies and takes legal action on specific issues. The membership group publishes the highly regarded and well-written *Environmental Action* magazine, started by the organizers of the *first* Earth Day. We can all be grateful that there are people like Ruth Caplan out fighting for the environment. Membership: $20, includes *Environmental Action* magazine.

ENVIRONMENTAL DEFENSE FUND, 257 Park Avenue South, New York, NY 10010, (800) CALL-EDF; FAX: (212) 505-2375, Executive Director: Frederic D. Krupp. Founded in 1967, this 150,000-member organization links the scientific, legal, and economic communities to create innovative, economically viable solutions to environmental problems. EDF is recognized as a tough, businesslike environmental group. Its staff of lawyers, scientists, and economists develop class-action suits and prosecute environmental offenders. As long as there are groups like EDF, those concerned with the environment will be able to sleep better at night. Membership: $20, includes bimonthly newsletter.

FOOD FIRST, 145 Ninth Street, San Francisco, CA 94103, (415) 864-8555; FAX: (415) 864-3909, Executive Director: Frances Moore Lappé. Founded in 1975, this outspoken organization of 20,000 members focuses on research and education regarding the empowerment of individuals to effect democracy at the grassroots level. They publish books that examine the root causes of hunger and powerlessness. They offer a free catalog of publications, including Lappé's extraordinary best-seller, *Diet for a Small Planet*. Ms. Lappé is one of the pioneers in this area, a totally devoted individual, deserving of the highest praise.

FRIENDS OF THE EARTH, 218 D Street, SE, Washington, D.C. 20003, (202) 544-2600; FAX: (202) 543-4710, Executive Director: Michael S. Clark. Friends of the Earth was founded in 1969 and recently merged with the Oceanic Society and the Environmental Policy Institute. The new group has 50,000 members and 37 international affiliates. It works locally, nationally, and internationally to protect the planet, preserve diversity, and empower individuals. It is an advocacy organization with lobbying function and it produces several publications. Membership: $25, includes *Not Man Apart* newsmagazine.

GLOBAL TOMORROW COALITION, 1325 G Street, NW, Suite 915, Washington, D.C. 20005-3014, (202) 628-4016; FAX: (202) 628-4018, President: Don Lesh; Vice President: Diane Lowrie. Founded in 1981, this association is an alliance of over a hundred member organizations that include some of the largest environmental and related-issue groups in the U.S. GTC acts as a clearinghouse for information and as an international liaison group. It conducts public forums and conferences (Globescope assemblies) and publishes and disseminates impressive and useful reports and guides at very low cost. It works to broaden public understanding of trends and their effects, and to promote global sustainable development. Membership: $35, includes newsletter and bulletins.

GREEN COMMITTEES OF CORRESPONDENCE, P.O. Box 30208, Kansas City, MO 64112, (816) 931-9366; Call for FAX number. Clearinghouse Coordinator: Jim Richmond. Founded in 1984, this organization is affiliated with the powerful international Green movement. This U.S. group is attempting to duplicate the political successes of European counterparts. The Greens have a highly developed, unified world view based on ten key values, ranging from the spiritual to the ecological. Listed here is the national information clearinghouse that will assist individuals in contacting one of the almost 200 local Green groups. Membership: $25, includes two quarterly newsletters, *Green Times* and *Green Synthesis*.

GREENHOUSE CRISIS FOUNDATION, 1130 Seventeenth Street, NW, Suite 630, Washington, D.C. 20036, (202) 466-2823;

Greenhouse Crisis Foundation (Continued)

FAX: (202) 429-9602, President: Jeremy Rifkin. GCF was formed in 1985 as a program of the Foundation on Economic Trends, a watchdog organization monitoring biotechnology research and regulation. The GCF disseminates information about global warming and the greenhouse effect. Global Greenhouse Network, a GCF project, is an international coalition to help facilitate global cooperation on the greenhouse crisis. GCF is funded by contributions and lecture fees. Jeremy Rifkin is as committed and dedicated a person as one will ever meet.

GREENPEACE, USA, 1436 U Street, NW, Washington, D.C. 20009, (202) 462-1177; FAX: (202) 462-4507, Executive Director: Peter Bahuoth. Founded in 1971, this is a nonviolent direct-action organization dedicated to preserving the earth and the life it supports. It works tirelessly to halt the slaughter of endangered species, to protect the environment from pollution, and to stop the threat of nuclear war. It is organizations like Greenpeace that keep hope alive that our children and grandchildren will have an environment that is whole and healthy. It has almost two million active supporters. Membership: $20, includes *Greenpeace* magazine, well worth the membership fee itself.

NATIONAL AUDUBON SOCIETY, 950 Third Avenue, New York, NY 10022, (212) 832-3200; FAX: (212) 593-6254, President: Peter A. A. Berle. Founded in 1886 by George Grinnel, this leading conservation group now includes over half a million members. It is dedicated to long-term protection and the intelligent use of wildlife, land, water, and other natural resources. It has lobbyists in Washington, manages 80 wildlife sanctuaries, conducts scientific field research, offers travel-study programs, produces outstanding television specials, and publishes several magazines, including *Audubon, Audubon Activist,* and *American Bird,* along with periodic Action Alerts. Membership: Introductory, $20, includes *Audubon* magazine.

NATIONAL WILDLIFE FEDERATION, 1400 Sixteenth Street, NW, Washington, D.C. 20036, (202) 797-6800; FAX: (202) 797-6646, President: Jay D. Hair. Founded in 1936, with the first North American

National Wildlife Federation (Continued)
Wildlife Conference convened by Franklin D. Roosevelt, its primary
objective is to promote the intelligent use of natural resources
through education, publications, and research activities. The nation's largest nonprofit conservation organization, it has almost six
million members and supporters. The NWF conducts investigations,
litigation and legislative campaigns, and publishes four magazines,
including two for children. Thanks to Jay Hair, the dynamic, dedicated president, the NWF has been transformed into one of the
leaders of the environmental movement in both the U.S. and the
world. Membership: $15, includes *National Wildlife* magazine.

NATURAL RESOURCES DEFENSE COUNCIL, 1350 New York
Avenue, NW, Suite 300, Washington, D.C. 20005, (202) 783-7800;
FAX: (202) 783-5917, Executive Director: John Adams. Incorporated
in 1969, the NRDC is a consumer-oriented watchdog group dedicated to protecting America's natural resources and improving the
quality of the human environment. It is due to the efforts of organizations like the NRDC that offenders of environmental laws are
made to toe the line. Its full-time staff of lawyers, scientists, and environmental specialists in four major cities combine legal action,
research, and education in their environmental protection programs.
It has 125,000 members. It publishes a newsletter and *Amicus Journal*
quarterly. Membership: $10, includes *Newsline* newsletter.

THE NATURE CONSERVANCY, 1815 North Lynn Street, Arling-
ton, VA 22209, (703) 841-5300; FAX: (703) 841-1283, President: Frank
D. Boren. Incorporated in 1951, with over half a million members,
this group works to find, protect, and maintain the best examples
of communities, ecosystems, and endangered species in the natural
world. Highly action-oriented, it is responsible for the protection of
almost four million acres of land in the Western Hemisphere. It has
created and maintains the largest private system of nature preserves
and habitats in the world (over 1000) and has current projects to save
200 key tropical areas of more than 100 million acres. The Conservancy also works in "debt-for-nature" swaps in South and Central
America. Speaking of debts, we all owe Frank Boren a debt—of gratitude. Membership: $15, includes *The Nature Conservancy Magazine*.

NEW FORESTS PROJECT, 731 Eighth Street, SE, Washington, D.C. 20003, (202) 547-3800; FAX: (202) 546-4784, Project Coordinator: Clifford Phillips. The NFP is a commission of the International Center for Development Policy, which sponsors delegations of prominent American officials and journalists to foreign countries. NFP sends information and tree seeds to forest-depleted areas worldwide. They sponsor regional training centers and seedling plantations, and produce a quarterly bulletin as well as brochures about specific tree species. Supported by foundation grant funding.

RAINFOREST ACTION NETWORK, 301 Broadway, Suite A, San Francisco, CA 94133, (415) 398-4404; FAX: 398-2732, Director: Randy Hayes. Founded in 1985, the work of this 25,000-member group includes highly active campaigns (even boycotts) to protect tropical rain forests in the U.S. and its Trust Territories, media campaigns, research on tropical timber and beef imports, and a worldwide directory of organizations working to protect rainforests. RAN produces *World Rainforest Report* quarterly magazine. Membership: $25, includes monthly newsletter.

RAINFOREST ALLIANCE, 270 Lafayette Street, Suite 512, New York, NY 10012, (212) 941-1900; FAX: (212) 941-4986, President: Daniel R. Katz. Founded in 1986, this 2,500-member group is committed solely to tropical forest conservation and the development of a national, broad-based constituency acting on their behalf. It works to educate the public and various professions about their interdependency with tropical forests and to facilitate their involvement. It also channels resources to local organizations in the tropics. Membership: $20, includes *The Canopy* newsletter.

RENEW AMERICA, 1400 Sixteenth Street, Suite 710, Washington, D.C. 20036, (202) 232-2252; FAX: (202) 232-2617, Executive Director: Tina Hobson. This group began in 1978 as the Center for Renewable Resources and The Solar Lobby. Several incarnations later, it is now Renew America, a 7,000-member organization. Their current mission is as an educational information network, involved with a coalition of environmental groups. They collect data and publish reports on various national issues with global implications. Their *State of the*

Renew America (Continued)
State annual report ranks all 50 states in 5 categories. Membership: $25, includes *State of the State* and quarterly newsletter, *Renew America Report*.

THE SIERRA CLUB, 730 Polk Street, San Francisco, CA 94109, (415) 776-2211; FAX: (415) 776-0350, President: Richard Cellarius. Since 1892, Sierra Club members (now numbering almost half a million) have lobbied to preserve national parks and wilderness areas and have worked for laws that ensure clean air and water. During that time, over a hundred million acres of wildlands and habitat have been protected. The focus of the Club is environmental action and outdoor adventure. It offers local, national, and international guided outings, member discounts, and local chapter membership. Membership: $33, includes *Sierra* magazine and chapter mailings.

TREES FOR LIFE, 1103 Jefferson, Wichita, KS 67203, (316) 263-7294; FAX: (316) 262-0211, Executive Director: Balbir S. Mathur. Founded in 1984, this group helps people in developing countries to plant and care for food-bearing trees. It acts as a catalyst for other groups, providing trees, management, and expertise. It has been responsible for the planting of millions of fruit trees in the Third World, and also provides "Grows-A-Tree" kits and materials for children in the U.S. at no charge. Any donation qualifies for mailings, and for copies of *Life Lines* newsletter.

THE TREE PEOPLE, 12601 Mulholland Drive, Beverly Hills, CA 90210, (818) 753-4600; FAX: (818) 753-4625, President: Andy Lipkis. Founded in 1973, this is an environmental problem-solving organization dedicated to promoting personal involvement, community action, and global awareness. With 7,000 members, it works with other organizations on projects, runs leadership programs for children, and assists community groups. It is responsible for the planting of millions of trees through education, information, and seedlings supply. This is an organization well deserving of your support. Membership: $25, includes *Seedling News* and six seedlings.

WILDERNESS SOCIETY, 1400 Eye Street, NW, Washington, D.C. 20005, (202) 842-3400; FAX: (202) 842-8756, President: George T. Frampton, Jr. Founded in 1935, this is the only national organization devoted exclusively to issues relating to preservation and management of wilderness and public lands of the U.S. It has vigorously fought misguided developers and bureaucrats, and is responsible for the Wilderness Act of 1964, establishing the National Wilderness Preservation system. This indefatigable lobbying group has 325,000 members and publishes the quarterly *Wilderness* magazine. Membership: Introductory, $15, includes *Wilderness* magazine.

WORLD HEALTH FOUNDATION FOR PEACE, 1400 Shattuck Avenue, Berkeley, CA 94709, (415) 783-7794, or: Bartolome de Las Casas 2273, Santiago, CHILE, 011 562-224-1144; FAX 011562-211-8442, President: Carlos Warter, M.D., Ph.D. Founded in 1982 by philosopher/author Carlos Warter, this organization is dedicated to the improvement of global understanding, ecology, education, and health, and its applications in science and technology, the arts, business, and government. WHFP functions as a link between like-minded individuals and groups in more than 40 countries, conducts international conferences and workshops, disseminates information, and actively promotes the concept of ethical, values-oriented leadership and the creation of optimum life quality. Membership by invitation. Further information available upon request.

WORLD RESOURCES INSTITUTE, 1709 New York Avenue, NW, Washington, D.C. 20006, (202) 638-6300; FAX: (202) 638-0036, President: James Gustave Speth. Founded in 1982, this is a policy research center dealing with environmental issues. WRI produces publications of which a list is available. The Institute is funded by foundation grants.

WORLDWATCH INSTITUTE, 1776 Massachusetts Avenue, NW, Washington, D.C. 20036, (202) 452-1999; FAX: (202) 296-7365, President: Lester R. Brown. Founded in 1974, this environmental research institute produces an array of highly respected publications. Its purpose is to inform policymakers and the public about the

Worldwatch Institute (Continued)
interdependence of the world economy and its environmental support systems. Its researchers analyze issues from a global perspective and its special reports are designed to fill the gaps left by more
specialized analyses. It offers a provocative but objectively edited
annual *State of the World* report, *World Watch* magazine and nearly 100
Worldwatch Papers to date, all of which supply the most factual and
up-to-date information on our planet's health available anywhere.
It is funded by grants and the sale of periodicals and reports.

ZERO POPULATION GROWTH, 1400 Sixteenth Street, NW, Suite
320, Washington, D.C. 20036, (202) 332-2200; FAX: (202) 332-2302,
Executive Director: Susan Weber. Founded in 1968, this 25,000-
member group promotes a sustainable balance among population,
resources, and the environment. It conducts advocacy activities and
offers teacher training. It distributes literature on national and global
population problems and policy responses; food and hunger; global
warming, and other related issues. Membership: $20, includes *ZPG
Reporter* monthly newsletter.

PUBLICATIONS

NOTES ON PUBLICATIONS
Most of the following are printed on all- or partially recycled paper. Several of the periodicals listed have pledged to plant at least one tree for every issue they publish, in accordance with the "Green Pages Campaign" instituted by *Earth Island Journal* (EIJ). Ultimately, they hope to replace the same number of trees that their publications consume. Contact EIJ for more information and a list of participating magazines. Additionally, the Australian magazine *Simply Living* is attempting to plant a tree for each new subscriber.

PERIODICALS INCLUDED WITH MEMBERSHIP DUES:
(These periodicals routinely include news pertaining to the organizations that publish them, but some have a broader range.)

AMERICAN FORESTS MAGAZINE, Published by American Forestry Association, Editor: Bill Rooney, Bimonthly; cover price: $2.50. Subtitled "The Magazine of Trees and Forests," it contains general conservation articles and related environmental information along with its major subjects: forests, urban and suburban trees in the U.S. and around the world. Exceptionally well edited and written; contains beautiful photographs.

EARTH ISLAND JOURNAL, Published by Earth Island Institute, Editor: Gar Smith, Quarterly; cover price: $3. Comprehensive reporting on global environmental issues, in news briefs and short pieces, with focus on "local news from around the world." Also includes several pages of EcoNet News (printouts from the EcoNet computer network).

ENVIRONMENTAL ACTION, Published by Environmental Action, Inc., Editors: Rosemarie L. Audette, Hawley Truax, Bimonthly. News, expose, resource guides, human-interest features, and citizen action alerts about waste and toxins, energy, and other issues. Especially targets national information.

GREENPEACE, Published by Greenpeace USA, Editor: Andre Carothers, Bimonthly; cover price: $1.50. Reports on Greenpeace action campaigns and ideas for action. Also contains articles on environmental issues and targets.

NATIONAL WILDLIFE, Published by The National Wildlife Foundation, Editor: Mark Wexler, Bimonthly. If you love critters, you'll adore the photographs in this publication. It's true to its name and contains interesting information about common and unusual species and their circumstances.

THE NATURE CONSERVANCY MAGAZINE, Published by The Nature Conservancy, Editor: Sue E. Dodge, Bimonthly. This house publication, available only to members, reports on land being acquired and species targeted for protection. It also includes articles about applicable issues and contains beautiful nature photography.

SIERRA, Published by The Sierra Club, Editor-in-Chief: Jonathan F. King, Bimonthly; cover price: $2.50. Features on conservation and other issues, articles on travel, hiking, and camping in wilderness areas, activist profiles, and information on Sierra Club outings. An outstanding example of top-flight writing and masterful photographic journalism.

WILDERNESS, Published by The Wilderness Society, Editor: T. H. Watkins, Quarterly. Gorgeous nature photography accompanies informative articles on preservation and protection of wilderness and wildlife. Not simple armchair travel fodder, this publication has visual appeal and substance.

THE FOLLOWING ARE PUBLISHED BY PREVIOUSLY LISTED ORGANIZATIONS, BUT ARE NOT OFFERED FREE WITH MEMBERSHIP:

THE AMICUS JOURNAL, Published by the Natural Resources Defense Council, Editor: Peter Borrelli, Quarterly; $10 annual subscription. An award-winning journal of thought and opinion on environmental affairs, especially relating to policies of national and international significance.

ORION NATURE QUARTERLY, Published by the Myrin Institute in association with Conservation International, Editor-in-Chief: George K. Russell, Quarterly; $14 annually or $4 each. Explores the relationship between nature and human culture, with a global focus. Includes essays, interviews, fiction, and an astounding array of photographic art features. Each issue has a major environmental theme.

WORLD WATCH, Published by the Worldwatch Institute, Editor: Lester R. Brown, Bimonthly; $20 annually or $5 each. A collection of reprinted articles by highly respected authors. Its goal is to help reverse the trends now undermining the human condition, raise public awareness of threats, provide a global framework for organizations working on the issues, identify new issues, and provide fresh insights.

THE FOLLOWING ARE OFFERED BY PUBLISHERS
NOT PREVIOUSLY LISTED IN THE ORGANIZATIONS
SECTION:

THE ANIMALS' AGENDA, Animal Rights Network, Inc., 456 Monroe Turnpike, Monroe, CT 06468, (203) 452-0446, Editor: Kim Bartlett, Ten per year; $22 annually or $2.75 each. Subtitled *The Animal Rights Magazine*, it also calls itself "the international magazine of animal rights and ecology." Includes articles, information and news briefs about animals, nature, endangered species, animal research and experimentation, factory farming, vegetarianism, and related environmental issues.

THE ANIMALS' VOICE MAGAZINE, Compassion for Animals Foundation, P.O. Box 341347, Los Angeles, CA 90034, (213) 204-2323, Publisher: Gil Michaels, Editor-in-Chief: Laura Moretti, Bimonthly; $18 annually or $4 each. Eye-opening news coverage and articles about both the treatment and the defense of animals by humans. Also includes interviews with protectionists, animal rights leaders and others; poetry, fiction, art and philosophy pieces, as well as investigative reports on abuse.

BUZZWORM: *The Environmental Journal*, 1818 Sixteenth Street, Boulder, CO 80302, (303) 442-1969, Editor/Publisher: Joseph E. Daniel, Bimonthly; $18 annually or $3.50 each. The name is old Western slang for a rattlesnake—a very effective communicator, as the editors see it. Features a variety of material dedicated to exploring environmental consciousness, including wildlife, travel, indigenous cultures, reports on trends, product information, "Eco-Business and "Eco- Fiction."

E: THE ENVIRONMENTAL MAGAZINE, Earth Action Network, Inc., 28 Knight Street, Norwalk, CT 06851, (203) 854-5559, Bimonthly; $20 annually or $3 each, Editor/Publisher: Doug Moss. Created to act as a clearinghouse of information, news and commentary on general environmental issues and trends for the public at large, in sufficient depth to involve dedicated environmentalists.

E: The Environmental Magazine (Continued)
Reports on activities of various organizations and includes suggestions for individual action. Also profiles innovative people working for the environment. A definite must for your library.

ENVIRONMENT, Heldref Publications, 4000 Albemarle Street, NW, Washington, D.C. 20016, (800) 365-9753, Editor: Barbara Richman, Ten per year; $24 annually or $5 each. In its fourth decade of publication, the magazine offers objective appraisals of problem areas, news briefs and reviews of governmental, scientific, and institutional reports, written to be accessible to the general public as well as the specialist.

THE FUTURIST, 4916 St. Elmo Avenue, Bethesda, MD 20814, (301) 656-8274; FAX: (301) 951-0394, Editor: Edward Cornish, Bimonthly; $30 annually or $4.50 each. This publication, while not strictly environmentally focused, covers every subject from resources to health to demographics and economics. It reports trends and ideas, and it forecasts the future. It includes an environmental section and is concerned with all aspects of how people will live in the 21st century.

GARBAGE, Old-House Journal Corporation, 435 Ninth Street, Brooklyn, NY 11215, (800) 274-9909, Editor/Publisher: Patricia Poore, Bimonthly; $21 annually or $2.95 each. Subtitled *The Practical Journal for the Environment*, it contains environmental science reports, informational articles and guides to responsible consuming, practical alternatives and recycling. Lots of usable information "about where things come from and where they end up," and how to prevent them from ending up in the wrong places. A strong, reasoned voice for environmental ethics.

SOLSTICE, 310 East Main Street, #105, Charlottesville, VA 22901, (804) 979-4427, Publisher: Randolph Byrd, Editor: John David Mann, Monthly; $21 annually or $3 each. Subtitled *Perspectives on Health and the Environment*, this magazine also calls itself the Voice of Macrobiotics. It offers features on natural foods, wild foods, and a wide range of environmental and social issues, with a macrobiotic

Solstice (Continued)

perspective. This is a hybrid of two original publications: Solstice and Macromuse.

THE UTNE READER, 1624 Harmon Place, #330, Minneapolis, MN 55403, (612) 338-5040, Editor/Publisher: Eric Utne, Bimonthly; $18 annually or $4 each. An "alternative" *Reader's Digest*, this is a collection of reprints from other sources. The articles have a political, environmental, and ethical orientation. Utne seeks to print stories not well-covered in the mainstream press. They have approximately 300,000 readers. A highly readable and provocative journal, chock full of interesting facts, ideas, and good writing.

VEGETARIAN TIMES, P.O. Box 570, Oak Park, IL 60603, (800) 435-0715, Publisher: Paul Obis, Jr., R.N., Editor: Sally Cullen, Monthly; $24 annually or $2.95 each. A nationally distributed consumer magazine with a meatless focus. Includes articles about health and fitness, profiles, consumer information, recipes, self-care, and the relationship of these areas to the environment. Do yourself and your family a favor and subscribe.

THE FOLLOWING PERIODICALS ARE PUBLISHED OUTSIDE THE UNITED STATES:

(Note: prices listed in foreign currency must be converted to dollars at current exchange rates.)

THE ECOLOGIST, Ecosystems Ltd., Corner House, Station Road, Sturminster, Newton, Dorset, ENGLAND, (02) 547-3476; FAX: (02) 587-3748, Editors: Edward Goldsmith, et al., Bimonthly; $30 annually (U.S.) or $6 each. A serious, somewhat academic, but very informative British magazine dealing with global concerns. Special issues treat one topic, deeply examined—for example, Amazonia. The papers and articles are written by scholars and environmentalists from the U.K., the U.S. and other countries, and are often footnoted with references.

THE ENVIRONMENTAL DIGEST, 3 Fernshaw Road, London, SW 100TB, ENGLAND, (0840) 212 711, Editor: Alex Goldsmith, Monthly; $20 (U.K.). A 12-page digest offering reprints of news of interest to environmentalists from British journals and newspapers.

SIMPLY LIVING, Otter Publications Pty Ltd., 46-54 Foster Street, Third Floor, Surry Hills, New South Wales 2010, AUSTRALIA, (02) 281-3784; FAX: (02) 281-4154, Publisher: Philip Kier, Editor: Samantha Trenoweth, Bimonthly; $45 annually (Australian) or $5.50 each. With over a quarter of a million readers, this is the country's journal of "modern environmental issues and ways of living, with Geographic-style nature photography." A quality magazine deserving of American readership. It is subtitled A Healthy Way to a Sound Environment.

ALSO NOTEWORTHY:

ECONET NEWS, 3228 Sacramento Street, San Francisco, CA 94115, (415) 932-0900. EcoNet is a computer-based communication system dedicated to helping the world environmental movement communicate more effectively. It is usually accessible through a local phone call (by computer modem) in the U.S. and in 70 foreign countries. It offers 80 public conferences in which users can read valuable information on a wide variety of topics. Users can also contribute information in response to others or as new topics. Private conferences can be set up for select numbers of users, for event-planning or collaborative writing. Subscriptions: $10 sign-up and $10 per month (applicable to one free hour of off-peak computer time). Off-peak time: $5/hour; Peak time: $10/hour.

THE WORKBOOK, P.O. Box 4524, Albuquerque, NM 87106, Subscription: $12 annually. This is a quarterly 125-page catalog of sources of information on social, environmental, and consumer publications.

RECOMMENDED BOOKS:

Berger, John J. *Restoring the Earth: How Americans Are Working to Renew Our Damaged Environment.* New York: Anchor Press, 1987. 241 pp., paperback, $9.95. Encouragement by example. This is a compendium of positive actions taken by Americans to conserve natural resources, wilderness areas, and endangered animals.

Brown, Lester R., et al. *State of the World 1990.* A Worldwatch Institute Report on Progress Toward a Sustainable Society. New York: W. W. Norton, 1990. 256 pp., paperback, $9.95. Published annually, this outstanding report is an in-depth assessment of world resources and management. It covers issues related to environment, population, and development and includes policy prescriptions and educated, feasible solutions for the world's most pressing problems. Must reading for informed citizens and every governmental official who has a vote on environmental matters.

Caufield, Catherine. *In the Rainforest.* Chicago: University of Chicago Press, 1984. 304 pp., paperback, $11.95. Not a "coffee-table book," this is scientific journalism at its best . . . a complete rain forest education: where they are, what they are, why we need them, and what's happening to them. Subtitled *Report from a Strange, Beautiful, Imperiled World,* Caufield went everywhere and spoke with everyone and came up with the goods . . . an outstanding job of research, reporting, and understanding. An unforgettable reading experience.

The Earth Works Group. *50 Simple Things You Can Do to Save the Earth.* Berkeley: Earthworks Press, 1989. 96 pp., paperback, $4.95. A wonderful guide that reads like a cross between *Ripley's Believe It or Not* and *Maryellen's Household Hints,* it is chock full of useful,

The Earth Works Group (Continued)
practical, and interesting information, as well as hundreds of impressive statistics for your ecological armamentarium. Simple, yes . . . but that is its virtue and its power as an important book for people who care, but feel they are too busy to do enough to make a difference.

Ehrlich, Anne H. and **Paul R. Ehrlich.** *Earth*. New York: Franklin Watts, 1987. 258 pp., hardcover, $19.95. This book examines the history of human interaction with the environment, and the nature, substance, and level of changes over time.

Fukuoka, Masanobu. *The Road Back to Nature: Regaining the Paradise Lost*. Tokyo and New York: Japan Publications, Inc., 1987. 377 pp., hardcover, $17.95. The author is the renowned microbiologist and plant pathologist who rebelled against the unnatural notions of modern agricultural science. He embraces farming as a spiritual path and has developed a practice of natural farming about which he has lectured internationally and written best-selling books. This is a collection of his impressions gathered while traveling across the world, observing man's despoiling of the earth. His ideas are worth heeding if we are to reverse the ecological disasters of desertification, deforestation, and destructive farming. Wisdom and readability you will treasure.

Global Tomorrow Coalition: *Citizen's Guide to Sustainable Development*. Washington, D.C. 1989. 350 pp., paperback, $5 from GTC. Beginning with a comprehensive overview of the current environmental situation, this information-packed guide thoroughly examines factors contributing to environmental degradation and their interrelationships, and suggests priorities, strategies, and personal actions. It contains extensive reference and resource material including charts, tables, graphs, and listings.

Goldsmith, Edward and **Nicholas Hildyard** (eds). *The Earth Report: The Essential Guide to Global Ecological Issues*. Los Angeles: Price Stern Sloan, 1988. 240 pp., paperback, $12.95. Compiled by two of the Editors of The Ecologist magazine (U.K.), this guide is organized in

Goldsmith, Edward (Continued)

two sections. The first is a collection of essays on a wide range of environmental issues. The second and larger section is an environmental primer with alphabetized data—facts, figures, terminology, concepts—from Acid Rain to Zero Population Growth. Illustrated with superior charts, graphs, and photographs. An important contribution.

Hollender, Jeffrey. *How to Make the World a Better Place.* New York: Quill, 1990. 303 pp., paperback, $9.95. This guide has three subtitles: *How You Can Effect Positive Social Change, Over 100 Quick-and-Easy Actions,* and *A Guide For Doing Good.* The 124 actions are grouped in six category chapters. Each has background information, including facts and figures, many of which are footnoted. It also has excellent resource and reference material. A book that lives up to its promise . . . loaded with useful information and ideas.

Lappé, Frances Moore. *Diet for a Small Planet.* Tenth Anniversary Revised Edition. New York: Ballantine Books, 1982. 469 pp., paperback, $11.95. The best-selling seminal work about changing diet and eating style to benefit the environment and also help curb world hunger problems. Includes dietary guidelines, preparation tips, recipes, and resource listings. A must addition to one's personal library.

Mason, Jim and **Peter Singer.** *Animal Factories.* New York: Crown, 1980. 174 pp., hardcover, $10.95. A courageous, eye-opening indictment and examination of America's "Agribusiness;" a shocking insight into mass production of animals for food . . . and how it affects the lives of consumers, farmers, and the animals themselves. Vividly illustrated with photographs, it also includes information about additives, disease, and consumer and farmer action toward improved methods. A landmark book.

Myers, Norman (ed). *Gaia: An Atlas of Planet Management.* Garden City, New York: Anchor Press, 1984. 272 pp., paperback, $18.95. Very comprehensive and supported by excellent graphics, this is a collection of pieces by an international group of environmental

Myers, Norman (Continued)
experts on a broad spectrum of issues, including social and political influences and implications.

Perlin, John. *A Forest Journey*. New York: W. W. Norton, 1989. 445 pp., hardcover, $19.95. A brilliantly conceived overview of five thousand years of man's dependence upon wood, the effects of that dependency on the world's forests, and the role forests have played in the development of civilization. Acclaimed by literary and environmental experts as the best book on the subject . . . comprehensive, clear, and very readable. A superb example of publishing excellence in every respect. Read it and you will weep for our disappearing forests.

Rifkin, Jeremy. *ENTROPY: Into the Greenhouse World*. New York: Bantam New Age, 1989. 354 pp., paperback, $12.95. A new edition of the environmental classic . . . serious, profound, and powerfully written. The author explains the universal concept of entropy, the tendency to move from an ordered to a disordered state, and how this law applies to the ecological crises threatening the earth. Using this model, he describes current trends and suggests a new world view based on an entropic model and a possible transition to a Solar Age.

Robbins, John. *Diet for a New America*. Walpole, NH: Stillpoint Publishing, 1987. 423 pp., paperback, $12.95. Written with passion and understanding, this powerful book exposes the inhumane treatment of animals raised as food and explores the connection of dietary habits to environmental conditions, as well as to health. A life-changing book that has been hailed as a masterpiece and has been compared to *Silent Spring* in its conscience-raising impact upon readers.

Schneider, Stephen H. *Global Warming: Are We Entering the Greenhouse Century?* San Francisco: Sierra Club Books, 1989. 317 pp., hardcover, $18.95. All about global warming. The book examines the causes, probable consequences, and possible remedies. Schneider, the action-oriented head of the Interdisciplinary Climate Systems

Schneider, Stephen H. (Continued)
Section of the National Center for Atmospheric Research in Boulder, Colorado, has written more than 100 papers on climate change, human impact on climate, and the climatic effects of nuclear war. This book is one of the clearest, most complete scientific assessments of climate change yet written for the general public.

Seymour, John and **Herbert Girardet.** *Blueprint for a Green Planet: Your Practical Guide to Restoring the World's Environment.* New York: Prentice Hall, 1987. 192 pp., paperback, $17.95. An exceptional work of reporting and publishing. The authors spent over two years traversing the globe for a BBC television series. The book offers hundreds of easy-to-use ideas for contributing to environmental restoration and includes excellent charts, graphics, and photographs. No library on this subject would be complete without this book.

The World Commission on Environment and Development. *Our Common Future.* New York: Oxford University Press, 1987. 383 pp., paperback, $10.95. Headed by Norway's Prime Minister Gro Harlem Brundtland, the World Commission was established by the United Nations in 1983 to define environmental issues and create a global agenda for change. People from all over the world spoke at its public hearings. In 1987, the commission (an impressive group of high-ranking officials and scholars) published this report, agreeing on the analysis and recommendations toward sustainable development. The book has three parts: Common Concerns, Common Challenges, and Common Endeavors. Required reading for global citizenship.

INDEX

A

Abbey, Edward, 123
Acid rain, 87
Agriculture, U.S. Dept. of, 40, 85, 124
Air, 91–99, 152
American Cancer Society, 27
American Forestry Association,
    173, 175–76
American Heart Association, 20
Animal products, 17–30, 46, 75,
    99, 107, 128, 142, 158, 159, 164,
    166, 179, 192; industry, 47–50,
    53–74, 77, 81–89, 160
Asimov, Isaac, 102
Atherosclerosis, 11–20, 107, 143

B

Biocides, 86
Biodegradable products, 183
Brower, David, 162
Browne, Jackson, 194
Brown, Lester, 40, 154
Bureau of Land Management, 124,
    125–26
Burke, Edmund, 155
Bush, George, President, 184

C

Carbohydrates, 28, 88

Carbon dioxide, 31–33, 48, 92–99,
    108, 109, 112, 147, 170, 171,
    173, 174, 182, 184
Cardiovascular disease, 11–20, 27,
    46
Carlyle, Thomas, 192
Carpooling, 182
Chlorofluorocarbons (CFCs), 70,
    185, 190
Cholesterol, 15, 17, 21, 24–26,
    28–29
Commoner, Barry, Dr., 162
Composting, trash, 186
Council on Economic Priorities,
    189
Council on Environmental Qual-
    ity, 121, 122
Cultural Survival, 113

D

Dairy products, 21, 76; industry,
    68
Deforestation, 87, 98–99, 110, 190
"Desertification," 120–123, 134
Dregne, Harold, 121
Drought, 33, 38, 40, 78

E

Earth Island Institute, 162
Ehrlich, Paul, Dr., 102